A DECADE OF LUPUS

Selected Articles from
LUPUS NEWS

Written and edited by
Henrietta Aladjem

Published under the auspices of
THE LUPUS FOUNDATION OF AMERICA, INC.

A DECADE OF LUPUS
SELECTIONS FROM LUPUS NEWS

HENRIETTA ALADJEM

LUPUS FOUNDATION OF AMERICA, INC.
4 Research Place, Suite 180,
Rockville, M.D. 20850-3226

Books by Henrietta Aladjem
The Sun Is My Enemy, 1972
Lupus - Hope Through Understanding –
Monograph on Lupus
Understanding Lupus, 1985
In Search of the Sun – Co-author
Dr. Peter H. Schur, M.D., 1988

Library of Congress Cataloging in Publication Data

ISBN-0-9608660-9-4

Printed in the United States of America

Typography and Printing, Acme Printing Company,
Wilmington, Massachusetts

This book is dedicated to Dr. Sergio Finzi, President Emeritus,
Lupus Foundation of America, Inc.

The first edition of 5,000 copies of this tenth anniversary
publication will be printed under the auspices of LFA. All
proceeds from this edition will benefit the LFA.

Disclaimer
The opinions and statements expressed by the authors
or contributors to this publication do not necessarily reflect
the opinions or positions of *Lupus News*, the LFA, Inc. or the Editor.

Editor

TABLE OF CONTENTS

CHAPTER 6
DOCTOR PATIENT RELATIONSHIPS

CHAPTER 7
MORE RESEARCH ON LUPUS

CHAPTER 8
LUPUS AND THE GOVERNMENT

DEDICATION*

To Dr. Sergio Finzi, President Emeritus of the L.F.A.

A DECADE OF LUPUS is dedicated to Dr. Sergio Finzi in recognition for his uniquely meritorious service to the LFA in the Office of President. Dr. Finzi has provided experienced leadership and expert management on a voluntary basis. His contributions to LFA's endeavors have been in giving of himself in terms of time, energy, effectiveness, and personal and material resources.*

*Excerpted from a talk given by Dr. Sheldon G. Cohen during the presentation of the LFA's Distinguished Public Service Award to Dr. Sergio Finzi in 1985.

ACKNOWLEDGEMENTS

A *Decade of Lupus* is written for the lupus patients and their families, for nurses and social workers, and all health care professionals. It is also written for the media and for the general reader who wants to know more about Systemic Lupus Erythematosus.

A Decade of Lupus is based on selected articles written for *Lupus News* over the past ten years. These articles are meant to bring hope and a better understanding of lupus from the physician's and patient's perspective. Hope based on facts is an important ingredient in sustaining the emotional balance of the patient. Norman Cousins once said: "If just the disease is treated without respect for the emotional state produced by the disease, you are only treating half of the patient." (quote from memory)

We are fortunate to have so many medical investigators and clinicians who have lent us their time, and their knowledge to make the writing of this book possible. We hope that *A Decade of Lupus* will raise the expectations of the patients and their hopes for a better tomorrow, perhaps even envision a cure for lupus in our lifetime. *A Decade of Lupus* is based on articles published in *Lupus News* over the past ten years. The choice of articles has been my own. This was a difficult choice! Many more articles could have been included in this publication. However, they were left out because of the size of this publication. Hopefully, some will be included in the next edition.

One cannot speak about *A Decade of Lupus* without stressing the many individuals who have helped and guided me to edit and write *Lupus News*. Dr. Peter H. Schur, Dr. Malcolm P. Rogers, and Dr. Arthur H. Krieg as Associate Editors have given a great deal of their knowledge and their time to make *Lupus News* the informative and educational paper it has become over the past ten years. The members of the Advisory Board and the Medical Advisory Board have also spent many hours making suggestions that arise from their sound medical, legal, and personal experiences. My heartfelt thanks to each and everyone.

I feel grateful to Ginger Ladd, immediate Past President of LFA, and our Board of Directors for entrusting me to write *A*

Decade of Lupus. And I must also thank John Walsh for faithfully distributing *Lupus News* to all the chapters over the past ten years and for keeping everyone happy and content. Our thanks go also to the Massachusetts chapter for their contribution of $10,000 to assure its continuous publication of *Lupus News*, and there have been other chapters around the country that have supported *Lupus News* in a similar way.

Many volunteers and professional typists have typed and retyped *A Decade of Lupus* and we thank them all for a job well done. And I must thank my steady group of young volunteers for proofreading the manuscript time and time again. To Vicki Croke, Donna McDermott, Susan Sepenuk, Krystyna Lulka, Nancy Connors, and Nancy Strisik many, many thanks.

And finally, I must express my love and gratitude to my twelve year old grandaughter Elise who likes to write like her grandmother. Elise spends hours by my side writing about her own fairy tale world, a world where we have all been at one time or another. Elise like all my other grandchildren answers the telephone, the doorbell, and does the small chores around the house, whenever I feel exhausted from writing another book about Lupus.

The Lupus Foundation of America and I want to express our gratitude to Susan Golick and the SLE Foundation of New York, a chapter of the LFA, for donating $10,500 to cover the printing expenses of *A Decade of Lupus*. Many thanks Susan!!! We also want to thank Jeanine Mingos and the Greater Washington Chapter for contributing an additional $2,500 to cover the typing, photostating and other incidentals. Our thanks to you too, Jeanine!!! We also want to acknowledge Acme Printing Company in Wilmington, MA, for their cooperation and special thanks to Fran Presti-Fazio, Dan Roden and Nelson Cohen. (Acme printed the first edition of *Lupus – Hope Through Understanding*, before it was taken over by Scribner's Sons in New York and won the Rodale Book Club Selection.)

LIST OF CONTRIBUTORS

Chester Alper, M.D., Professor of Pediatrics, Harvard Medical School; and Scientific Director, Center for Blood Research, Boston, MA.

Stanley P. Ballou, M.D., Associate Professor of Medicine Case, Western Reserve University of MetroHealth Medical Center, Cleveland, OH.

Yves Borel, M.D., Associate Professor of Pediatrics, Harvard University Medical School, Director, Rheumatology Services, Children's Medical Center, Boston, MA.

Otis Bowen, M.D., Former Secretary of Health and Human Services, Washington, D.C.

Ronald I. Carr, M.D., Ph.D., Division of Rheumatology, Halifax Civic Hospital, Halifax, Nova Scotia.

Laszlo Czirjak, M.D., Ph.D., Third Department of Medicine University Medical School of Debrecen, Debrecen, Hungary.

Venus Dartez, Executive Secretary Public Information Office, Oklahoma City, OK.

Judah A. Denburg, M.D., FRCP(C) Professor Department of Medicine, Director Lupus Clinic, Head Clinical Immunology and Allergy, McMaster University, Hamilton, Ontario, Canada.

Jeramie Dreyfuss, Patient, Hollywood, CA.

Luis Fernandez-Herlihy, M.D., Head of Rheumatology, Emeritus, Lahey Clinic, Burlington, MA., Former Lecturer Harvard University Medical School.

Robert F. Garry, Ph.D., Associate Professor, Department of Microbiology and Immunology, Tulane University School of Medicine, New Orleans, LA.

Jeffrey P. Gilbard, M.D., Clinical Assistant Professor, Harvard University Medical School, Clinical Associate Scientist, Eye Research Institute, Massachusetts Eye & Ear Infirmary Boston, MA.

Monica Gilliam, R.N. and Lupus Patient, Detroit, MI.

Ming Jiang, M.D., Peking Union Medical College Hospital, Institute of Basic Medical Sciences, Chinese Academy of Medical Sciences, Beijing, People's Republic of China.

John H. Klippel, M.D., Clinical Director, National Institute of Arthritis and Musculoskeletal and Skin Diseases, Bethesda, MD.

Arthur M. Krieg, M.D., Assistant Professor of Medicine, University of Iowa, Iowa City, IA.

Robert G. Lahita, M.D., Ph.D., Assistant Professor of Medicine, Columbia University, Chief of Rheumatology, St. Luke's - Roosevelt Medical Center, New York, NY.

Moe Liss, President, Lupus Foundation of New Jersey.

Daniel Magilavy, M.D., Associate Professor of Medicine and Chairman, Section of Rheumatology, University of Chicago, LaRabida - University of Chicago Institute, Chicago, IL.

Gale McCarty, M.D., FACR, Associate Professor of Medicine, Oklahoma University Health Science Center and Medical Research, Oklahoma City, OK.

Alan Metzger, M.D., Associate Clinical Professor of Medicine, UCLA, Clinical Chief Division of Rheumatology, Adar Mount Sinai Medical Center, Los Angeles, CA.

John D. Reveille, M.D., Associate Professor, Department of Rheumatology, University of Texas, Health Science Center, Houston Medical School, Houston, TX.

Malcolm P. Rogers, M.D., Psychiatrist, Assistant Professor of Psychiatry Harvard University Medical School; Division of Psychiatry, Brigham and Women's Hospital, Boston, MA.

Everett Newton Rottenberg, M.D., P.C., F.A.C.P., Clinical Associate Professor, Wayne State Medical School, Detroit, MI.

Peter A. Schur, M.D., Professor of Medicine, Harvard University Medical School, Director Lupus Research, Senior Physician, Brigham and Women's Hospital, Boston, MA.

Robert S. Schwartz, M.D., Professor of Medicine, Tufts University Medical School; Director, Cancer Research, and Chief of Hematology, New England Medical Center, Boston, MA.

Jean Luc-Senécal, M.D., FRCP, Associate Professor of Medicine, Director Rheumatology - Immunology Research Labs and Connective Tissue Disease Clinic, Division of Rheumatology, Notre-Dame Hospital, Montreal, Quebec, Canada.

Howard S. Shapiro, M.D., Assistant Clinical Professor of Psychiatry, University of Southern California School of Medicine, Los Angeles, CA.

Emilia Spassova, M.D., Plovdiv, Bulgaria.

Louis W. Sullivan, M.D., Secretary of Health and Human Services, Washington, D.C.

Jane Tado, Director of Federated Programs, L.F.A.

Stephen E. Ulrich, Ph.D., Assistant Professor, Department of Immunology, The University of Texas, Anderson Cancer Center, Houston, TX.

M.B. Urowitz, M.D., FRCP, Professor of Medicine, University of Toronto, Physician-in-Chief, Wellesley Hospital, Director Lupus Clinic, Wellesley Hospital, Toronto, Ontario, Canada.

Daniel J. Wallace, M.D., F.A.C.P., F.A.C.A. Diplomate, American Boards of Internal Medicine and Rheumatology, Los Angeles, CA.

Laurie C. Williams, A Patient, Baltimore, MD.

Liping Zhu, Ph.D., Peking Union Medical College Hospital, Institute of Basic Medical Sciences, Chinese Academy of Medical Sciences, Beijing, People's Republic of China.

INTRODUCTION

This collection of articles was selected from ten years of writings which appeared in *Lupus News*, the official Newsletter of the Lupus Foundation of America. Most of them were written by physicians from a wide range of different specialties, but all with a common interest in lupus and lupus patients. Frequently they were written in response to specific questions from patients and their families so that they could cope more effectively with their disease. The articles convey not only information that may illuminate previously puzzling aspects of lupus, but, equally important, the limits of that knowledge, and the efforts to expand it, so that new therapies can be found.

Articles by patients also offer a crucial dimension in this compilation celebrating the tenth anniversary of *Lupus News*. They inform doctors and other care-givers about the true meaning of illness. Each illness experience binds the patient's unique personal history and aspirations for the future, with a particular set of biological disruptions brought on by the disease. The physician's job is to relieve suffering, which requires not only diagnosis, and biological intervention, such as medicines but equally skillful psychological intervention, such as listening, understanding and providing hope.

Even if they could, not all lupus patients would choose to read this book. Some would prefer to remain ignorant of the details, preferring to leave that to their doctors to worry about. It's not a bad strategy when it works. It frees patients to focus on their own lives and activities (apart from the illness) in the larger community. It would work better if the disease were brief in duration, and could be fixed by surgery or a single course of chemotherapy. The problem with lupus is that, once present, it remains a continuing presence, or at least a potential threat. Typically, it comes and goes, and in many different ways, visible or invisible, sudden or gradual, so as to escape notice. Like it or not, patients are forced to be participants in a lengthy process of identifying symptoms, taking medicines, modifying important life decisions such as child bearing, and interacting with the health care system. Faced with this challenge, an informed participant is likely to have a less frustrating experience over the long haul than an uninformed one.

Similar foundations have come to exist for most diseases to provide information and group support to patients and to raise money for research. The Lupus Foundation was among the first. Henrietta Aladjem has led the way, turning her singular talents for communication and writing to the subject of lupus and disseminating it throughout the world.

There are an estimated 500,000 Lupus patients in this country, and certainly a much greater number throughout the world. In consolidating these articles from the last 10 years of *Lupus News*, Mrs. Aladjem has once again found a way of reaching out to them all.

Malcolm P. Rogers, M.D.

1

An Overview of Lupus

John H. Klippel, M.D.

Images perhaps better than words are a good place to start an introduction about lupus. The images are all personal ones of patients and their families who have struggled with the disease. Most involve fear evident on the faces of patients or even shared by a trembling, crying 10 year old who with a hug says "I'm scared". The fear is of illness, real or threatened, and what lupus will do to their lives. Often the fear is replaced by the joy of overcoming the disease — the medical student who recovers after months in the hospital, returns to school, graduates, starts her own career, marries and gives birth to a daughter. In others the outcome is far sadder — the task of telling parents and a young man engaged to be married that a young girl has unexpectedly died from lupus is not something ever forgotten.

This book is written for people who wish to learn more about lupus — patients, their families and loved ones, and health care professionals who are faced with the challenge of trying to help patients who suffer from the disease. The overview and writings that follow provide a small glimpse of lupus as seen from the eyes of many people who have tried to better understand this mysterious illness.

History Of Lupus

The use of the term lupus, Latin for wolf, to describe diseases associated with skin rashes dates to medieval times. Very accurate descriptions and pictures of the common rashes seen in lupus patients can be found in medical writings throughout the nineteenth century. Towards the latter part of the century a number of prominent physicians particularly Moritz Kaposi in Vienna and Sir William Osler from the Johns Hopkins Hospital in Baltimore are credited with recognition of the potential serious nature of the disease. The ability of lupus to affect the joints, lymph glands, heart and lungs, kidneys, abdominal organs, or brain was well documented. However, major advances in drug treatment of the disease and insights as to the cause of lupus were not discovered until the late

1940's. The observation that corticosteroid hormones produced dramatic improvements in the clinical manifestations of lupus and other rheumatic diseases resulted in the award of the Nobel Prize in Medicine in 1950 to Dr. Philip Hench and Dr. Edward Kendall from the Mayo Clinic and Dr. Tadeus Reichstein of Switzerland. The discovery of the LE cell by Hargraves, Richmond and Morton also from the Mayo Clinic revealed for the first time disturbances of the immune system in patients with lupus. The factor responsible for the LE cell was found to be an antibody to the nucleus of the cell, the antinuclear antibody. For the last four decades, the primary focus of research in lupus has been aimed at efforts to understand what causes the immune system to produce these abnormal antibodies.

Epidemiology

Studies done throughout the world have found that lupus is a reasonably common disease (Table 1). Interestingly, the studies confirm the impression that lupus is increased in certain racial groups particularly black individuals, chinese, and polynesian populations. The highest prevalence of the disease reported to date comes from a study done in San Francisco with the finding lupus may be as common as 1 in every 250 black females. These studies suggest the important of inherited factors and the apparent increased occurrence of genes associated with lupus in select populations.

Although lupus may affect people of either sex or occur at any age, young females are clearly at greatest risk for the development of the disease. The ratio of females to males with lupus is in the range of 10 to 1. It is believed that the influences of female sex hormones, particularly estrogens, on the immune system make females more susceptible to the development of lupus. Additional evidence to support this interpretation include the development or worsening of lupus with pregnancy or with the use of birth control pills, instances in which estrogen levels are increased.

Clinical Signs And Symptoms Of Lupus

The clinical signs and symptoms of lupus can be divided into general, non-specific illness (systemic or constitutional signs), non life-threatening clinical manifestations (skin rashes, mouth ulcers, arthritis, and serositis) or potentially serious involvement of major organs (heart, lungs, kidneys, or brain).

Systemic or Constitutional Signs

Most lupus patients simply don't feel well. The symptoms are often quite vague — unexplained fevers, poor appetite, weight loss, weakness, nausea, emotional changes, or the inability to concentrate or think clearly. Complaints of being tired all the time or lacking energy (fatigue) are particularly common. Patients wake up in the morning with no energy or become so exhausted during the day that they are simply not able to function. In some patients specific causes for these complaints such as anemia, infection or involvement of the kidneys or brain can be found. In many patients, however, no abnormalities to explain the symptoms can be found — a situation equally frustrating to both the patient and the physician.

Skin Rashes

Skin rashes are extremely common in patients with lupus. Rashes on the cheeks, or to use the medical term malar rashes from the latin *mala* meaning cheeks, are perhaps the best known clinical sign of the disease. Malar rashes often appear suddenly and are typically intensely red (erythematosus). The rash may affect the entire surface of the cheeks or develop as many small, measles-like blotches. The rash often extends across the bridge of the nose (the well known butterfly rash) or may spread to involve the forehead or chin. A fine scaling of the skin often develops at the borders of the rash. The intensity and redness of the rash gradually fades over several days or weeks typically leaving no trace of damage. Similar rashes may develop on the upper part of the chest, the arms, and the backs of the hands and fingers. Curiously, lupus rashes on the fingers develop in a very characteristic location of the skin areas between the joints themselves.

Discoid rash refers to a very different form of skin involvement that may occur as an isolated skin condition (discoid lupus) or as part of systemic lupus erythematosus. The discoid eruption typically begins as multiple small red spots (plaques) covered with a whitish scale. As the rash expands, the area in the center becomes depressed and often loses normal skin pigment whereas the expanding border of the rash continues to show redness and thickening of the skin. Characteristic locations of discoid rashes include the face, neck, ears, arms, and upper part of the chest. The scalp is a common site of discoid involvement and may be associated with permanent hair loss. There are several important differences between malar or erythematosus rashes and discoid rashes; the two most important of which are that discoid rashes are often painful or associated with itching and may produce extensive scarring and disfigurement.

The development or worsening of lupus rashes by sunlight (photosensitivity) is a rather characteristic feature of most lupus rashes. The distribution of lupus rashes primarily on the face, upper part of the chest, arms, and back of the hands likely results from the exposure of these areas to sunlight. In some patients, other forms of light such as ultraviolet light rays in tanning parlors or even overhead fluorescent lights are capable of adversely affecting lupus rashes. In some patients who are highly sensitive to light, severe exacerbations of lupus, including internal organ involvement, can be caused by light exposure.

Arthritis

Arthritis is the first manifestation of illness in roughly one-half of lupus patients. In the absence of other findings, it may be very difficult to distinguish lupus arthritis from other causes of joint disease, particularly rheumatoid arthritis. Although any joint may be involved, knees, wrists, and the small joints of the hands are most commonly affected. Symptoms such as pain or joint stiffness are often prominent in the morning and may occur without noticeable changes in the joints such as swelling or redness. The arthritis often tends to migrate from one joint to another and rarely lasts longer than several days in any individual joint. Although lupus arthritis is not associated with destructive changes of bone or cartilage on x-rays, patients with recurrent arthritis may develop joint deformities that result from loosening of the tendons and ligaments that support the joints. The deforming arthritis most commonly occurs in the hands and may be responsible for significant limitations of hand function. Persistent joint pain, particularly in the hips, knees, shoulders, or ankles, may be a sign of other joint complications such as infection or avascular necrosis of bone (see Corticosteroids).

Mouth Ulcers

Ulcers may form on the roof of the mouth or mucous membranes surfaces of the cheeks. Similar lesions may develop on other mucous membrance surfaces including the inside of the nose, surfaces of the vagina, or lining of the rectum. Typically, the ulcerations don't cause pain although they may be associated with bleeding or become infected.

Serositis

Lupus may produce inflammation of the membrances that line the lungs (pleuritis), the heart (pericarditis) or the abdomen (abdominal serositis). This may cause excruciating chest or abdominal pain that may be confused with a heart attack or appendicitis. On physical examination, abnormal sounds (rubs) may be heard through a stethoscope or a collection of fluid (effusion or ascites) may be found. Methods used to document serositis include x-rays, ultrasound, electrocardiogram, or the removal of fluid through a needle.

Kidney Disease

Involvement of the kidneys in lupus is referred to as lupus nephritis or lupus glomerulonephritis. These are few signs or symptoms to alert a patient as to the presence of kidney disease. The retention of fluid with weight gain or ankle or leg swelling (edema) particularly at the end of the day may be noticed by the patient. Studies performed on urine and blood are critical in the identification of kidney involvement in lupus (see Laboratory Studies). In patients with obvious evidence of kidney disease, a kidney biopsy may be needed to confirm the diagnosis or determine the extent and severity of the kidney involvement to help in making decisions about treatment. The specimen obtained by kidney biopsy is examined for increases in the numbers and types of cells present in the kidney (proliferation), abnormal thickening in the walls of the kidney vessels, or any scarring that may have developed. Based on these findings, a reasonable estimate of the seriousness of lupus nephritis can be made. In many patients, the abnormalities found are mild and may require little or only minor changes in therapy. However, in other patients, more serious abnormalities associated with an increased risk of continued kidney damage and loss of kidney function are found that require major changes in drug therapy.

Heart and Lungs

Involvement of the heart or lungs in patients with lupus are both uncommon. On examination of the heart, murmurs from abnormal growths of the heart valves are often detected (Libman-Sacks endocarditis). Although these rarely, if ever, produce symptoms, patients with murmurs may require antibiotic treatment with dental or other surgical procedures to prevent the development of infections on the damaged heart valve. Recently, it has become recognized that lupus patients are at increased risk for the development of coronary atherosclerosis that may produce angina pectoris or myocardial infarction. It remains to be determined whether this results from the underlying lupus itself or is secondary to other factors such as hypertension, kidney disease, or drugs used in treatment.

Cough, shortness of breath, or chest pain often of acute onset may be clues to several different forms of lung involvement seen in patients with lupus. Inflammation developing within the lung tissue may result from lupus (lupus pneumonitis) or occur secondary to an infectious process. Distinguishing between the two is often difficult, yet important, since infectious complications require prompt treatment with antibiotics. In addition, certain patients with lupus are at increased risk for blood clots to the lungs (pulmonary emboli).

Neurologic Disease

Neurologic involvement in lupus can produce an assortment of symptoms depending on the structure of the nervous system affected by the disease. Involvement of the brain, or central nervous system lupus, is most common. This may cause neurologic injury such as seizures, paralysis of a limb, or impairments of sensation. In addition, psychiatric symptoms such as severe depression, emotional disturbances or thought abnormalities may develop. Involvement of the spinal cord (myelopathy) may result in the inability to move the arms or legs, decreased sensation of the extremities, or loss of bowel or bladder function.

Laboratory Studies

Laboratory studies are important to determine the effects of lupus on the kidneys, the bone marrow, and the immune system.

Evidence of lupus nephritis is typically identified by examination of a urine specimen (urinalysis) or by blood studies that measure levels of chemistries altered by disease of the kidney. Abnormalities that may be detected on urinalysis include protein in the urine (proteinuria), red blood cells (hematuria) or white blood cells. On examination of the urine under the microscope, the protein or cells may be clumped in the shape of the collecting tubules within the kidney (casts). Involvement of the kidney by lupus nephritis may impair the kidney's primary function to eliminate body waste products. Studies done on the blood measure levels of these waste products, particularly the blood urea nitrogen (BUN) and serum creatinine. In addition, the loss of protein in the urine may lead to reduced levels of proteins in the blood, typically measured by the level of serum albumin. The collection of urine over a 24 hour period allows for more sensitive measurements of both protein loss in the urine and level of kidney function (creatinine clearance).

A complete blood count (CBC) is used to evaluate the effects of lupus on the bone marrow. Essentially all three of the primary blood cell types formed in the bone marrow may be affected in patients with lupus. Reductions in red blood cells (anemia) may result in fatigue, pallor, or shortness of breath. Reductions in white blood cells (leucopenia) may be associated with an increased risk of infection. And reductions in platelets (thrombocytopenia) may cause increased bruising or bleeding. The reductions in these blood cell types may result from the direct effects of lupus on the bone marrow or involve the rapid destruction of the cells by antibodies formed against outer membranes surfaces of the cells.

The major laboratory hallmarks of lupus are antibodies that react with structures of the normal cell, so-called autoantibodies. In particular, antibodies against parts of the cell nucleus (antinuclear antibodies) are of considerable importance and can be identified in essentially all patients with the disease. More specific types of antinuclear antibodies such as antibodies to deoxyribonucleic acid (anti-DNA) or antibodies to the Smith antigen (Sm) are almost unique to the disease. Antinuclear antibodies are very important in diagnosis and changing titers of antibodies are frequently used to follow the course of the disease.

Another type of antibody commonly found in lupus patients reacts with lipid (fatty) molecules on the surface of cells. The two types of these antibodies that are commonly measured are the anticardiolipin and antiphospholipid antibodies. These antibodies are responsible for the positive syphilis tests often seen in lupus patients. In addition, these antibodies are found frequently in lupus patients who experience certain complications of the disease such as thrombophlebitis, thrombocytopenia, neurologic disorders, or recurrent abortions.

The measurement of complement levels in the blood is helpful in determining ongoing damage from lupus. As a consequence of immune-medicated injury, for instance an antinuclear antibody affixing to the kidney in a patient with lupus, complement proteins automatically become deposited within the area of damage. Thus the levels of complement with the blood may become reduced when lupus is active and return to normal when the immune injury has resolved. Common measurements of complement include C3, C4 and total hemolytic complement (CH 50).

Diagnosis

The diagnosis of lupus typically requires that both clinical and laboratory evidence of the disease are present. The patient who presents with classic signs and symptoms such as a butterfly rash, arthritis, pleurisy, and kidney disease who on laboratory testing is found to have a positive antinuclear antibody, antibodies to DNA and low levels of complement is readily diagnosed with the disease. However, if the clinical signs and symptoms develop over many months or even years, it may be much less apparent that lupus is the cause of the illness. For instance, in the evaluation of a patient with unexplained nephritis, neither the patient nor the physician may recognize that the one week history of arthritis 5 years earlier and the brief episode of pleurisy two years ago are in fact important clues to the diagnosis. Thus in these types of patients there are often long delays before the correct diagnosis is made. Similarly, the patient with one or two signs of lupus such as arthritis and positive antinuclear antibody presents an equally difficult problem. Although in general the possibility of lupus is often considered, the diagnosis can't really be made with certainty and an effective plan of treatment is by necessity often delayed.

Research

The autoantibodies identified in lupus patients are regarded as central to the disease process. Examination of the organs affected in lupus reveals a concentration of these antibodies that are thought to be responsible for the inflammation that is produced. This gives rise to the concept that lupus is an antibody-mediated, systemic inflammatory disorder. What causes the antibodies to be formed in the first place and why they then become deposited in tissues become the major important research questions in understanding the disease.

The two primary factors that are thought to be important in the production of autoantibodies are environmental agents and genetic factors of the patient. In all likelihood, these are mutually dependent on one another for autoantibodies to develop. For instance, a person would need exactly the right combination of genes and contact with a particular environmental agent for autoantibodies to be formed. Several lines of evidence would seem to support this notion. For example, certain drugs (environmental agents) are capable of producing antinuclear antibodies, as well as clinical symptoms of lupus. Conceivably, there are as yet unidentified environmental agents (toxins or allergens, food substances, infectious agents, etc.) that are responsible for lupus. Moreover, it is entirely possible that there may not be a single cause of the disease but rather multiple different responsible agents. The evidence for the importance of genetic influences are several — an increased frequency of lupus in identical twins and in certain families with lupus, the increased occurrence of the disease in racial groups, and the identification of certain HLA genes associated with the disease.

The other major question in lupus involves why the antibodies that are formed then go on to produce clinical disease. There would seem to be the potential for problems at several different levels. First under normal circumstances, the immune system regulates or shuts off the production of antibodies. In lupus patients this regulatory function appears to be impaired resulting in the uncontrolled production of excessive quantities of antibodies. Secondly once the antibodies are released into the blood circulation, excess quantities of the antibody are removed or cleared from the circulation by the so-called reticuloendothelial system made up of organs like the spleen and liver. Some lupus patients have a marked decreased ability to clear these antibodies. This may be related to defective signals to detect the antibody or simply the massive quantities of antibody present simply far exceed the capacity of the reticuloendothelial system to remove them. The overproduction of antibodies combined with the failure to adequately clear them results in high antibody levels detected in the blood of lupus patients. These antibodies are then thought to become deposited in multiple tissues where they ordinarily don't belong such as the skin, kidneys, lungs, etc. to set off an inflammatory reaction and produce the clinical signs and symptoms seen in patients with lupus.

Management

General principles that are important in the management of patients with lupus would include the following:

Regular Physician Visits Irregardless of the health of the lupus patient, regular physician visits are extremely important. The types of physicians who commonly care for lupus patients include specialists in internal medicine, rheumatologists, and immunologists. Physicians with expertise in the management of specific problems that develop in lupus patients may be involved in health care such as nephrologists for kidney disease, neurologists or psychiatrists for central nervous system involvement, or orthopedic surgeons for surgical management of serious, destructive arthritis. The frequency of physician visits may be as often as daily or weekly in the patient with evolving signs or symptoms or as infrequently as yearly in the patient who is entirely well and in remission. The purposes of the visits are many — physical examination and blood and urine tests to detect evidence of lupus problems, adjustments of drug therapy, or monitoring for toxicities from the drugs used in treatment.

Photoprotection Patients who are sensitive to the sun or other forms of light must remember to minimize intense sun exposure. This includes adjustment of activities to avoid daylight hours of peak sun intensity (10 a.m. to 4 p.m.), the liberal use of sunscreen lotions, and the wearing of appropriate clothing to reduce sun exposure — long pants, long sleeve blouses, or large-brimmed hats.

Infection Control Infections are increased in patients with lupus and are a frequent cause of serious illness requiring hospitalization. Unexplained fever, chills, or sweats may be signs of an underlying infection and require prompt evaluation by a physician. Several measures can be taken to reduce the risks of infection including immunizations with vaccines such as yearly flu shots or pneumococcal vaccine in patients who have had their spleens removed. Patients who are undergoing dental or surgical procedures in which there is a risk of infection should receive antibiotics at the time of the surgery.

Pregnancy Issues Since the majority of lupus patients are young females, there are several issues relating to pregnancy. Birth control is particularly important in the lupus patient with major, serious organ involvement from the disease or when certain chemotherapy drugs are used in treatment (see below). In lupus patients who are pregnant there are potential risks to both the mother and the developing fetus. For the mother, there is a small risk of worsening of the lupus during pregnancy. Thus, more frequent visits to the physician including blood and urine tests to detect any changes in the disease are essential. In addition, obstetrical care for the baby is generally provided by physicians with expertise in the management of high-risk pregnancies. It is particularly important that the primary care lupus doctor and obstetrician work closely together throughout the pregnancy to assure the health of both the mother and the baby.

Drug Therapy

Drugs are an important part of management in some patients with lupus. Several different classes of drugs are used depending on both the type and severity of lupus manifestation being treated. Some of the more common drugs used in the treatment of lupus patients are discussed below. In addition, however, it is important to recognize the valuable role of drugs in the treatment of various complications that may develop in lupus patients such as anti-hypertensive drugs for high blood pressure, diuretics for fluid retention, antibiotics for infections, or anticonvulsants for seizure disorders.

Antiinflammatory Drugs

Drugs that reduce the level of inflammation (antiinflammatory drugs) have an important role in the treatment of symptoms such as fever, arthritis, and fatigue. Both common medications such as aspirin or drugs containing Ibuprofen (Advil®,

Nuprin®, Medipren®, and others.) as well as drugs available only with a prescription (Naprosyn®, Feldene®, Orudis®, and many others) are used. Individual patients may be respond better to one drug than another so that often several different medications may need to be tried before the ideal drug is found. The most common side effect of this group of drugs is gastrointestinal complaints such as nausea, vomiting, or stomach pain. Taking medications along with food or the use of antacids often relieves these symptoms. Serious complications from these drugs are rare but include bleeding from the gastrointestinal tract, skin rashes, hepatitis, fluid retention, and meningitis.

Corticosteroids

Of all the drugs used in the treatment of lupus, corticosteroids are unquestionably the most important. Corticosteroids may be used as pills (prednisone, etc) or given by injections or intravenous infusions in patients with more serious manifestations of the disease. In addition, creams that contain corticosteroids are useful in the management of lupus rashes. Most patients have rather prompt and often dramatic improvement in the disease after corticosteroids are started. The selection of the dose of corticosteroid to be used is extremely important since the risks of side effects increases with higher doses of the drug. In general, the decision as to the corticosteroid dose is based on the seriousness of the disease. For instance, problems such as arthritis, rashes, fatigue, or mild pleurisy ordinarily improve with low-doses of corticosteroids with little risk of complications. On the other hand, serious manifestations such as kidney involvement or central nervous system disease may require higher drug doses associated with a far greater likelihood of a complication. Once lupus is under control with corticosteroids, the dose of corticosteroids is slowly reduced (tapered) and the patient carefully monitored for signs of recurrence of lupus. In general, the goal is to reduce the corticosteroid dose to the lowest dose possible that controls symptoms. Many physicians will attempt to change the patient to an alternate day corticosteroid schedule to minimize the risks of complications.

Corticosteroids are natural hormones produced by the adrenal glands located above the kidneys. It is extremely important to recognize that corticosteroid hormones are essential factors required to maintain a normal state of health. One of the consequences of many months of corticosteroid use is the shrinkage of the glands that naturally produce cortisone. The glands may in fact eventually cease to function and fail to produce corticosteroid hormones on their own. The patient therefore becomes entirely dependent on corticosteroid drugs for the hormone. Thus, patients who have been on corticosteroids for many months or years must remember the absolute importance of taking corticosteroids as directed. The abrupt discontinuation of corticosteroids can be extremely dangerous and lead to serious illness. In emergency situations, it is extremely important that rescue and hospital staff be aware that the patient is under treatment with corticosteroids. Thus, many patients wisely elect to wear Medical Alert bracelets containing information as to the fact that the patient has lupus and the drugs used to treat the disease.

There are a number of potential side effects of corticosteroids. Both the dose of corticosteroids and how long they are used are important factors in the risks of the side effects. Most obvious are changes in appearance with weight gain, fullness in the cheeks, and the development of stretch marks or bruises on the skin. The resistance to infection becomes lowered with increases in minor skin, respiratory, and urinary tract infections as well as more serious infections. The effects of corticosteroids on bone may lead to a process called avascular necrosis (osteonecrosis) or a reduction in the mineral content of bones or osteoporosis. Avascular necrosis is a potential complication following high dose corticosteroid use and may result in a serious form of arthritis typically involving large joints such as the hips, knees, and shoulders. Other possible complications of corticosteroids include high blood pressure, diabetes, and cataracts.

Antimalarials

Drugs used in the treatment of malaria are often valuable in the management of certain symptoms of lupus including fever, fatigue, arthritis, and in particular skin rashes. Of the antimalarial drugs, hydroxychloroquine (Plaquenil®) given in low doses is by far the most widely used. The use of hydroxychloroquine is generally regarded as quite safe and associated with few side effects; gastrointestinal complaints and occasional skin rashes are perhaps most common. Much attention has been focused on the potential toxicity of the drug to the retina of the eye. Fortunately, serious eye complications from low-dose antimalarial use are extremely rare. As a precaution, however, patients treated with antimalarials should have a careful eye examination at least yearly to detect any early evidence of damage to the retina from the drug.

Investigational therapies

Several approaches to lupus management involve drug therapies or procedures that would be regarded as investigational. In certain instances, evidence from research studies would indicate that the therapies are in fact effective such that they have become widely used in lupus management.

Considerable interest in drug therapy of lupus has focused on drugs that suppress the function of the immune system. The drugs most commonly used for this purpose include cyclophosphamide (Cytoxan®), chlorambucil (Leukeran®), and azathioprine (Imuran®). In general, these drugs are reserved for patients with serious manifestations of lupus such as advanced kidney disease or central nervous system disease. The reduction in functioning of the immune system caused by the drugs produces an increase in the risk of infection. Careful monitoring of the white blood cell count and adjustment of drug dosage are extremely important to reduce the risk of infection. Other potential side effects of immunosuppressive chemotherapies include hepatitis from azathioprine and hair loss, bleeding from the urinary bladder, and sterility from cyclophosphamide. In addition, immunosuppressive drugs may produce birth defects and are contraindicated in pregnancy. Thus birth control measures are extremely important in patients who are being treated with these drugs. Finally, there is reason to suspect that immunosuppressive drugs may increase the risk for the development of cancer.

Additional investigational approaches to lupus management that involve alterations of the immune system include plasmapheresis and radiation therapy. Plasmapheresis is based on the theory that abnormal antibodies with the blood are responsible for the clinical signs and symptoms of lupus. Removal of the plasma, or liquid phase of the blood, might then be expected to result in improvement in the disease. Although plasmapheresis has been the subject of several research studies in lupus over the past decade, there is still considerable controversy as to the effectiveness of this approach. Recently, a large international study to examine the effects of plasmapheresis combined with cyclophosphamide has been organized by investigators in Kiel, West Germany. This important study will provide additional information as to the role of plasmapheresis in lupus. Radiation therapy to the primary organs of the immune system (total lymphoid irradiation) produces suppressive effects on immune function similar to chemotherapy. Radiation has been used with reported favorable results in a small number of patients with lupus kidney disease. Further studies involving this experimental approach are currently in progress.

Table 1.   Studies of prevalence of systemic lupus erythematosus.

	Cases/100,000
United States	
San Francisco, CA	51
Black	168
Oahu, HI	
White	6
Hawaiian	20
Japanese	18
Rochester, MN	40
New Zealand	
Auckland	18
White	15
Polynesian	51
Dunedin	23
China	
Shanghai	70

2

A Few Words About
Dr. Sergio Finzi, Ph.D.

D r. Sergio Finzi, prior to becoming the President of the Lupus Foundation of America, led an incredibly productive and exciting life. As Assistant to the President of a pharmaceutical company in Ecuador during the late 1940's, Dr. Finzi served as the firm's "troubleshooter." He was actively involved in every phase of the business.

After leaving the latin american company, Dr. Finzi spent 30 years with Schering Corporation. But one thing didn't change. He was still actively involved in every phase of the business.

By heritage, temperament, and training, Dr. Finzi was well prepared to help lead a relatively small company, as Schering Corporation was during the early 1950's, from its domestic orientation into the demanding world of multinational ethical pharmaceutical corporations.

Dr. Finzi was born and reared in Venice. His family had been successful Venetian traders and bankers for generations.

Dr. Finzi's personality was attuned to the fast-paced, rigorous tempo of international management in which government decisions, currency fluctuations, and competitors' strategies can unravel months, even years, of careful planning in days — and new opportunities appear just as quickly. Dr. Finzi always seemed comfortable with this intense environment, which seems in harmony with his own drive and determination.

Dr. Finzi is also a perfectionist. He was told years ago that he could take up fishing to relax. "In no time," a colleague noted, "he was pursuing fishing with the same discipline and energy he exhibits in other activities. Sergio is determined to excel in anything he undertakes, and now fishing is among his greatest pleasures."

Soon after his graduation from the Italian Institute of Economic Sciences with a doctor of economics degree, Dr. Finzi and other members of his family became targets of racial harassment on the eve of World War II. In 1939, therefore, he left Italy for Paris, where he hoped to join a company owned by a friend of his father. Unable to obtain a resident permit in

France, however, Dr. Finzi went to Brussels, where he pursued additional studies.

But with typical Finzi persistence, he returned to Paris. This time Dr. Finzi took part in a major trade fair as an expert in techniques for extracting oil from grape seeds, an industry with which his family had long been familiar. But his application for a resident permit was again denied. After a brief trip back to Italy, Dr. Finzi departed for London.

In late 1941, Dr. Finzi booked passage to South America despite World War II naval disruptions and dangers. After a brief delay in Argentina, he reached Ecuador and was soon involved in his uncle's business.

The war ended. Dr. Finzi briefly returned to Italy but decided not to stay, in light of political and economic uncertainty in his native country to which he still returns frequently to visit his brother and sister. He again left for Ecuador and soon joined a pharmaceutical company employing about 500 people in Quito, with branches in Central America, Colombia, and Venezuela. Dr. Finzi was named Assistant to the President.

During a trip to the United States in December 1950, Dr. Finzi met Joan Newman, a fashion coordinator for an advertising agency, who was living in New York. A week later, he asked her to marry him; and the following March, she flew to Ecuador for their April wedding. But the couple soon began planning to settle permanently in the United States.

Dr. Finzi joined Schering Corporation in 1951 as an international sales correspondent responsible for Ecuador and Colombia — countries with which he was very familiar, of course. Soon he was handling the company's sales throughout Latin America.

For more than 20 years, Dr. Finzi's career had primarily focused on the Western Hemisphere. But with Schering's new regional organization, he returned to Europe as director of the new Region II office in Milan, responsible for Europe, the Middle East, and Africa. Dr. Finzi was prepared for this challenging assignment through his years as International Division marketing manager, his European business heritage, and his fluency in English, French, Italian, Portuguese, and Spanish. In 1966, he was named an International Division Vice President.

"As all of us knew, this region had extraordinary potential," Dr. Finzi said. "But in 1962, Schering sales there were only $2 million in U.S. We had a lot of work to do."

During the next decade, Schering's presence spread throughout Europe and in many Middle Eastern and African countries as well. The infrastructure of organizations, facilities, and people for which Dr. Finzi and other company managers had aimed took shape.

By 1970, Schering's yearly business in Europe, the Middle East, and Africa had increased to more than $50 million U.S. Dr. Finzi was appointed Corporate Vice President for international operations the same year and returned to Kenilworth, N.J.

After his long, fast-paced career, few colleagues can imagine Dr. Finzi pursuing a traditional, leisurely retirement. He can't either. "It's my intention to dedicate most of my time to the Lupus Foundation of America, a patient-oriented organization pursuing support for research into the causes of this terrible and little understood disease," said. Dr. Finzi.

Systemic lupus erythematosus is an elusive disorder which is often misdiagnosed as rheumatoid arthritis. It appears to make the body "allergic" to some of its own tissue and most commonly afflicts women between the ages of 15 and 40. Although lupus is less well known than leukemia, multiple sclerosis, and muscular dystrophy, it is more common and just as serious.

3

Dr. Walter Heller
Remembered, 1915-1987

Regents' Professor Emeritus Walter W. Heller, advisor to Presidents Kennedy and Johnson, combined his knowledge of economics with his ability to communicate to become one of the best-known economists in the country, an outstanding professor at the University of Minnesota, and a major contributor to modern economic policy-making.

Dr. Heller went to Washington in 1961 as Chairman of President John F. Kennedy's Council of Economic Advisers. Dr. Heller was one of the architects of the "War on Poverty" programs that were enacted under President Johnson. Heller believed in using government policy to change the course of the nation's economy. He was proud that his economic policies improved life for the poor.

Walter Heller called himself a child of the Depression. The thought of learning the causes of the Depression and trying to do something about them was what attracted him to economics. The son of immigrant german parents, he received his bachelor's degree from Oberlin College, in Ohio, and his master's and Ph. D. degrees from the University of Wisconsin.

Dr. Heller's wife of 47 years, Emily, whom he called "Johnnie," died in 1985 after a 25-year battle with lupus. The Hellers helped to streamline the Lupus Foundation of America and fought, with the rest of us, to bring public awareness of this still little-known disease.

The Hellers are survived by their daughter Karen Heller Davis, of Seattle; two sons, Eric, a Professor of Chemistry and Physics at the University of Washington, and Walter P., a Professor of Economics at the University of California at San Diego; and six grandchildren.

When asked about his career just prior to his retirement, Heller said, "I'm just one of those lucky people who's been given an opportunity to do what I wanted to do — a life in academia, teaching, and public service. Luck has to play a role."

At a memorial service for Walter Heller, his colleagues and

friends turned out at the University of Minnesota, on Friday, June 26, 1987, to remember this wonderful man. The speakers were:

— Harlan Cleveland, Professor and Dean, Humphrey Institute, University of Minnesota
— Kenneth H. Keller, President, University of Minnesota
— Walter Mondale, Vice President of the United States and former Senator from Minnesota
— Atherton Bean, former Chairman and CEO, International Multifoods
— James Tobin, Sterling Professor of Economics, Yale University Nobel laureate, Economics
— N.J. Simler, Professor and Chair, Economics, University of Minnesota
— George Perry, Senior Fellow, Brookings Institution; former Professor of Economics, University of Minnesota
— Geri Joseph, Senior Fellow, Humphrey Institute, University of Minnesota
— Hobart Rowan, Economic Columnist, *Washington Post*
— Leo Hurwicz, Regents' Professor of Economics, University of Minnesota
— Henrietta Aladjem, personal friend of Walter and Johnnie Heller. Worked closely with Walter and Johnnie through the Lupus Foundation
— Phil Raup, Professor Emeritus, agricultural and applied economics, University of Minnesota
— William G. Shepard, Professor Emeritus, Electrical Engineering; former Vice President, University of Minnesota
— Walter P. Heller, Professor of Economics, University of California at San Diego

Washington Post, Economics Columnist, Hobart Rowan remarked, "Walter educated not only Kennedy and Johnson but a whole generation of journalists like myself."

Walter Mondale, Vice President of the United States and former Senator from Minnesota, said, "Kennedy is gone, and Hubert is gone, now Heller is gone, and it hurts. But you also have the sense that what Heller did will endure."

Senator Edward M. Kennedy was quoted as saying, "When you were in a room with Walter Heller, economics was never a dismal science but a fascinating public discipline, alive with possibilities for hope and progress."

Dr. Sergio Finzi, Past President of the LFA, commented, "Dr.

Walter Heller will be remembered by many in a variety of ways. My recollections of him stem from our working together as volunteers for the Lupus Foundation. Busy as Dr. Heller was with his teaching and his other involvements on the national and international scene, he always found the time to help us to promote the growth of the Lupus Foundation of America. Walter Heller contributed substantial personal funds to the Foundation; and as the chairperson of the National Campaign Committee, he generated additional monies for public awareness and education for this still little-known disease.

"Dr. Heller and I had a strong bond of purpose, for he and I understood firsthand the ravages of this disease — Dr. Heller, by losing his wife, Emily, to lupus; and I, by losing Gina, one of my two daughters. We shall all miss him."

*"The sudden death of Dr. Walter Heller has brought sadness and grief to all of us. His moral and financial support of public awareness and education of lupus has helped us to create a better understanding of what this illness can and does do to a human life. Dr. Heller had a love for humanity which was an outpouring of everything good in him — it was kindness and courage and hope for a better world for all.

"I was grateful for Walter's support for our work, and I was very glad and happy for it. I respected his friendship, and I tried to live up to it. I'll keep a picture of Emily and Walter in my heart, and I'll be looking at it for strength and inspiration.

"Emily and Walter have both departed to find themselves within the folds of nature. They are asleep under the huge maple trees at Beachwood on Hood Canal, where the ocean struck by the light of the stars seems to absorb their brightness.

"The place under the trees is marked by silence, mystery, and dreams — drifting out to us — but nevertheless, in saying farewell, I weep.

"I find it hard to articulate how much Emily and Walter Heller just meant to me — and to all of us. We shall miss their friendship."

*From the Eulogy read by Henrietta Aladjem at the Memorial Service for Dr. Walter Heller, at the University of Minnesota.

4

UNDERSTANDING THE CHALLENGES FOR THE LUPUS PATIENT FROM THE PATIENT'S PERSPECTIVE

Psychosocial Aspects of Rheumatic Disease – A Patient Speaks*

When I was first diagnosed as having systemic lupus erythematosus (SLE, or lupus), it was a frightening experience. I had never heard the word lupus before or known of anyone who had anything similar to what I had. I was told that I was suffering from a rare, mysterious disease that affects predominantly blue-eyed blonds with a pink complexion like mine.

At that time in the history of medicine (1953), lupus was considered uniformly fatal. When I didn't die, the physicians questioned the diagnosis.

On my own, all I could find out about the disease was that lupus comes from the Latin and it means *wolf;* and erythema, from the Greek, means literally to be red. The first thing that came to mind was — What does the wolf and lupus have in common? The question kept hammering away in my mind. The very sound of the disease was lethal because of identification with the predator.

Unfortunately, even today, patients read or hear that lupus is invariably a fatal illness; this leads to great anxiety. Similarly, a patient may be told that she or he has arthritis, which leads to ungrounded fears of disabling deformities. And physicians observe that, when one adds to these natural fears and anxieties a frank organic psychosis, one gets a hyperirritable, confused person who is afraid of living and afraid of dying.

Help with such fears requires much of the physician's time and a real understanding of the patient's stresses.

Lupus is no longer a rare disease, and it is far from being fatal. Physicians stress that the past few decades have been an exciting time for research regarding better understanding of the pathogenesis and pathophysiology of lupus. The medical community feels that today the major problems facing patients and physicians are those of chronic disease with both complications of the disease and therapy.

But do the physicians know what this disease does to a human life? Without knowing this, can they properly treat the patient?

To me, lupus remains a disease with a name that's difficult to pronounce and more difficult to live with. It is a disease with an unpredictable prognosis and symptoms that are difficult to explain. It is intermittent, recurrent, and it nibbles away at the will to live and the ability to cope. It can threaten life and it can prevent the patient from functioning like a normal human being.

I have spent many hours at medical libraries searching for literature on the psychosocial and emotional problems of the lupus patient. I found that such problems were rarely mentioned in the psychiatric literature; and when they are, focus is directed toward SLE with central nervous system involvement. I could not find anything to reflect the fears and apprehensions of the individual — of human suffering — the very core of the disease. In lupus, the body and the soul are enmeshed in a sense of pain and desperation that makes it difficult for the physicians to distinguish whether they are dealing with a neurotic who has developed lupus or a lupus patient who has developed a neurosis because of the disease. Some physicians say it is difficult to tell for sure in some patients. This makes one wonder whether many young women who are so-called neurotics do not have a touch of lupus.

Physicians often ask me, "When did your lupus begin?" There are so many beginnings, so many experiences, I never know how to explain the symptoms so that they won't judge me a fool. Looking into the distant past, I wonder whether the disease was inherited. In adolescence, my parents attributed some of my afflictions to a delicate constitution: constant strep throats, susceptibility to colds, recurring pneumonia, and the overreaction to mosquito bites. In my case, sunlight affected my skin. My skin needed protection from heat, cold, wind, ultraviolet light — anything that touched it. The rash that I got from the sun or the blue blotches from the cold induced parallel changes in my system. The skin reaction was more spectacular, while the reaction of the internal organs was more dangerous.

The drugs I took, instead of helping, caused more problems

that were rarely interpreted correctly. The reaction should have been perceived as a warning signal from nature, not just for one drug, but for all.

The patient with lupus is concerned not only with the immediate side effects of the drugs but also with side effects that may appear years after a specific drug was taken. Medications with well-established toxicities are frequently used in the management of this disease. This has evolved because of the frequency of a life-threatening situation or because the restrictions placed on the seriously ill patient become unacceptable to her and her family. The lupus patient remains a consumer of the most experimental nature.

Very often the drugs prescribed by the physician depend on which research center you go to and who is the attending physician.

The lupus patient is a bewildered human being who is besieged by physical, emotional, and economic problems. The patient becomes ruled by fears — fears that others will find out that one is struck by a mysterious illness, fear of being cut off from the human flow of life, fears of not being able to do the things one was trained to do. One gets worse and then gets better without obvious cause. And there are times when the patient is the only person who is sure that one is really sick but doesn't know what is wrong.

You try to tell the doctor about the transient nodules under your elbows, the migratory pains and aches, the inflammation that comes and goes unpredictably, particularly swelling and reddening of the soles of your feet that are present one day and by the next day may have disappeared. You watch the doctor's expression change from an attentive one to one of obvious annoyance, and there are moments when you begin to wonder whether what you are trying to tell him is even true.

The symptoms of the patient are often insidious, and they can confuse even the most knowledgeable physician.

Most lupus patients, if not all of them, experience an intense fatigue. The lupus fatigue is unique — it absorbs the whole person. It doesn't act like an organic, psychologic, or physiologic fatigue. It doesn't respond to drugs, rest and relaxation, or psychiatric help. You cannot call it malaise or even lethargy. You feel depleted of energy and spiritually exhausted, to the point where even brushing your teeth becomes a difficult chore. At times, the sense of futility is so great that one becomes tempted to "give up" or give in to permanent sleep. What keeps one going is the need to help one's children, attend to a job, or the moral responsibility one feels for life itself.

The lupus patients I know don't believe the physicians can even begin to imagine the physical and psychologic desperation created by the lupus fatigue.

The need for linking the lupus fatigue to our profound depression is becoming more and more urgent as observations reveal its damaging effect in many, and to a certain degree, perhaps in all. Many lupus patients describe this fatigue as their first symptom of lupus. They claim that they experience this symptom even when their physicians tell them that they are in remission.

Lupus is not just another chronic disease.

What makes it so difficult is that the symptoms come and go unpredictably, and the patient doesn't show any signs of deterioration. The people around you see you well one moment and distressed the next; and they can become distrustful and feel that you may be a hypochondriac or, even worse, a person who will always find excuses for poor performance.

When emphasis on neurosis is accentuated by the physician, it becomes destructive to the whole family because this implies that the person has control over this illness, which one absolutely does not.

And the patient makes the mistake of thinking that they are causing all the difficulties when it is really the illness.

In the early 1970s, the American Rheumatism Association established preliminary criteria for SLE based on the presence of four or more of fourteen manifestations. The criteria will be expanded as new information comes in. *Lupus fatigue should be placed high on the list.*

As for me, I was fortunate. I had good doctors; they cared and they wanted to help me. They stuck by me and gave me courage. We interacted as people. The physician became the *person* who could help me; and I, the *person* who needed to be helped. Even though I was told from the beginning that they didn't know of any cure, I was encouraged to believe that the will to live and the desire to cope were regenerating forces playing an important role in fighting lupus. In my case, what medical science could not do, the doctors achieved with their humanity.

For the past 15 years, I have been in complete remission. I have a checkup once a year, and I am on no medication. When patients ask me what am I doing to stay well, I tell them that I am a living example of Osler's aphorism: If you want to live a long life, get a chronic disease and learn how to take care of it. The secret is to reach and alter the whole way of life, by probing for and correcting all the various noxious influences — diet, medication, general hygiene, proper medical attention and rest; and we must learn to avoid stress to any extent possible.

And finally, when patients ask me whether I still take the nicotinamide, I tell them, yes, I do — for sentimental reasons. But I am realistic. I know that the predisposition to lupus will always be present, as well as the lack of resistance to infections, severe reactions to drugs; and the sun will always be my enemy.

And I would like to add a sentence in the words of Dr. Rene Dubos: "The hope in the future lies in the physician's willingness to listen to the patient, and the patient's courage to reject medical science without humanity."

*This Chapter was written by Henrietta Aladjem. It has appeared in the seventh edition of the PRIMER. It is reprinted with permission from the Arthritis Foundation, Atlanta, Georgia.

Jeramie Dreyfuss Testifies On Behalf of The LFA in Washington, D.C.

Jeramie Dreyfuss, wife of actor Richard Dreyfuss, testified before a Senate subcommittee on behalf of the Lupus Foundation of America. The Dreyfusses; Nancy Horn, President of the Los Angeles Chapter; Henrietta Aladjem, Chair of the Public Relations Committee; Cindy Carway; and staff members of our Washington office were cordially received by Senator Ted Kennedy, Senator Dole, Senator Childs, Senator Shelby, and Senator Weicker. The Senators listened to the grievances of people with lupus and the great need for increases in funding for biomedical research and lupus for the National Institutes of Health.

We also had appointments with other members of our government, such as Congressman Joseph Early, of Massachusetts, which we couldn't keep because of time constraints. We even had an appointment with Ms. Duggan, liaison for health with President Reagan. In the past, it was Mrs. Virginia Knauer at the White House with whom we worked closely and who was instrumental in helping the LFA to be included in the Combined Federal Campaign (CFC) program. We hope that in the future Ms. Duggan will help us with our public relations efforts so we can reach every person with lupus in the United States.

Mrs. Dreyfuss, who has lupus, captivated everybody in Washington with her outgoing disposition, sincerity, and charm. I have seldom seen a young woman who loves humanity with such passion as Jeramie does and who places children, especially suffering children, as one of her top priorities to love and to help. The Dreyfusses appeared on the Larry King Show. Their appearance on the show brought innumerable inquiries from persons with lupus to our national office.

Here is Jeramie's testimony as she presented it to the Senate subcommittee in D.C.

Good morning. My name is Jeramie Dreyfuss. I am a wife, a mother, and I have lupus. I'm here today on behalf of the Lupus Foundation of America to impress upon the urgent need to continue NIH support for biomedical research into the causes of and cure for lupus.

What I am recounting today is not the total of my medical history but only some of the misunderstood and puzzling episodes that no one could figure out for so long. Over the years, I've been hospitalized 28 times and operated on so often for so many different, seemingly unrelated, reasons that it is hard to keep an accurate count. Today, the reasons don't seem nearly as unrelated as they once did. Through advanced diagnostic and therapeutic methods that have brought about a deeper knowledge of lupus, we can now see a common thread running through each episode that I've experienced. That thread is the immune system and its failure to do its job properly.

At the age of 16, I nearly had a leg amputated for what appeared to be abnormal growths. I continued to have major medical problems with my leg that defied explanation.

At the age of 24, I underwent a three-vertebrae spinal fusion to alleviate mysterious and excruciating pain. The day following the surgery, I suffered an unbearable attack of pain in my abdomen. After an emergency appendectomy, they informed me that I had indeed had peritonitis, a potentially fatal inflammation of the abdominal cavity, but my appendix was fine. When I say potentially fatal, I mean that the condition has been known to kill its victims within hours of their developing it.

Four years later, I suffered five more such attacks. Each time the doctor could not explain it, each time the doctors said it was impossible. What that means is, peritonitis is caused by something but they could never figure out what that something was. That is not an unusual reaction for a lupus patient to experience, because with lupus the damage being done within the body is not always visible to the naked eye. I insisted they take a blood test. My fears were well founded. My white blood count had soared and the peritonitis had reoccurred. Massive antibiotics saved my life.

I was convinced I was going to die in 1978 from this unexplainable illness.

I was diagnosed with lupus in 1979. Knowing nothing about the disease, I searched out information at Cedars Sinai Hospital only to learn that I had a life expectancy of five yeears. That's what the medical experts believed about lupus in 1979.

Following the birth of my first child, I lost the use of both hands and arms due to a lupus flare that lasted two years. I eventually required surgery on both hands and my right shoulder.

That I am sitting here today is due in large measure to the fact that the American medical and scientific communities are the most advanced in the world. I was treated successfully and I am pulling through so far. But I am one of the lucky ones. I am considered to have a mild case.

I am here today on behalf of every one of the 500,000 Americans who have lupus. And, I am here today for the sake of my son and daughter. My daughter Emily, who is four years old, has already suffered one unexplained high white count called a leukemoid reaction. It terrifies me to think that she might have to suffer the way I have.

For the sake of the next generation, please help us fight diseases like lupus that so threaten the health of the American public. Only research can cure this disease — only your funding can give us that research. Thank you once again for this opportunity.

Letter On Denial of
Social Security Benefits

By Monica Gilliam, R.N., A Patient

Dear Editor,

The following is an excerpt from my response and request for reconsideration of my social security disability benefits:

To Social Security Administration (SSA):

Please direct your attention to the fact that since 1977 my disease has progressed, in spite of continuous treatment, at a somewhat rapid rate. Initially there were multiple arthralgias and decreased pulmonary function. Subsequent flares have caused further damage, consequently creating problems in terms of activities of daily living. Medical records confirm that I was hospitalized several times for exacerbations of SLE.

My rheumatologist considered adding anti-malarial drugs to my present course of therapy with the hope of halting the progression of the disease. However, such drugs are con-traindicated . . . I have extensive retinal damage.

It is a known fact among SLE patients that regardless of laboratory findings, most of the time we feel quite sick, lack energy, have joint pains, muscle pains, and experience great difficulty performing our duties, even simple personal care. These symptoms are intermittent and vary from day to day, sometimes even during the course of the same day. Only someone who sees me frequently can testify about my performance.

The medications which I must take for control of symptoms cause drowsiness and lethargy. As a nurse, I must be alert and able to perform whenever my patients need my services. Otherwise, I became a danger to the patients and increase the risk of legal liability on my part and that of the hospital for which I work.

My job also requires my driving to patients' homes at times to render nursing care and supervise others. At present, I am unable to drive myself for my therapy at the Rehabilitation Institute three times per week. Stair climbing is also difficult —

how can I serve these patients?

I have not asked to be placed on medical disability for an indefinite period. I could not live with that thought. My strength of will makes me believe that I will experience a remission. However, it is unlikely that a remission will be attained if I am forced to return to my job while I am still impaired. It is my perception that SSA is forcing me to work, without regard for my pains and other symptoms. I am simply requesting my prorated benefits until my health improves.

There are times when I am unable to hold a pan due to painful fingers and wrist, even when swelling is minimal. It is evident there are contractures of my hand. I need assistance getting dressed at times — even your doctors had to assist me when they performed the exams you demanded. You mentioned that according to my X-rays there's a lack of joint pathology. Please be informed that, unlike arthritis, SLE joint pains and weakness seem to be caused mainly by affected tendons, not bone degeneration.

I have cooperated and submitted to rather uncomfortable examinations on two occasions by doctors of your choice. The diagnosis has been confirmed. The degree of my symptoms vary. Presently I am very uncomfortable sitting, needless to mention walking, due to skin eruption.

Rejection by SSA has aggravated my situational depression because I (and persons who know me well) know that I love my work; therein lies my strength. I have put much effort into my career, and have written recognition to show. As soon as I am able, you will not need to force me to return. In 1978 I returned to work full-time under my own direction, not my doctors'. Even though I was not well, I was better and wanted to work. I still want to try, but I am having greater difficulty doing so at this time. Furthermore, my doctors advise much rest — I am told that rest is probably the most important therapy. You seem to be telling me to go against my physicians' advice.

Perhaps you may need to revise your protocol with assistance from systemic lupus erythematosus sufferers who can give you first-hand information about a disease which most experts in the field agree is an unpredictable, puzzling, incurable disease — a disease which requires much further research.

What is the Lupus Foundation of America doing to assist people who have been denied their Social Security benefits?

Letter on Minorities and Lupus

By Laurie C. Williams, A Patient

Dear Editor:

I am corresponding with you to express my appreciation for your informative and enlightening interview with Louis W. Sullivan, M.D., Secretary of Health and Human Services. As a 27-year-old African-American female and lupus patient, I was particularly pleased with the focus on the severity of lupus in the African-American community. I was diagnosed with lupus in 1984 while pregnant with my son. At that time, I was told that there was evidence of a higher incidence of lupus among black females, but additional information was scarce. Since then I have sought out as much information as possible concerning our disease, but I still feel at a loss. The *Lupus News* has been instrumental in providing 99% of the information available, however, Mrs. Aladjem, I feel it is not reaching the minority community. Special methods and considerations must be utilized in a stronger effort of inclusion of young African-American women in an active and highly visible role in the struggle for public awareness.

I grew up in a predominantly white community in Allentown, PA and attended a grade school with a majority of white, Jewish, upper-middle class students. However, my family moved to a more racially mixed community in Ravenna, Ohio, and I was fortunate to be able to reinforce my lost roots and culture during high school and college. I feel my life has been ideal in allowing me to be able to relate to whoever I meet. I can pick up any publication, whether it is *Lupus News, Goodhousekeeping*, or whatever, and benefit from the information enclosed no matter the point of view from which the story is told or the race of those individuals pictured. But as I've stated, my background has been ideal, and an exception rather than the rule for the majority of young black females in our society.

The statistics are clear. African-American mortality is at an all time high from all causes. Our society has desperately failed in providing medical education in the minority community. But what can be done? You asked Dr. Sullivan that question, and his answer was right on track. We must design educational materials and programs specifically aimed at minority audiences.

I am a wife and mother. I majored in journalism in college where I attended Bowling Green State University. I work part-time outside the home as a veterinary receptionist, but am currently pursuing a career as a freelance writer. I have battled my disease and weathered my crises as we all have, and that within itself I feel is a triumph. But I feel like I can and must do more. I would like to channel my energies to addressing the problem we have discussed. I would like to extend my hand to you, specifically Ms. Aladjem, as a tool for opening doors in our struggle for national attention that have consistently remained closed to minorities. I'm offering my help and assistance in whatever capacity to reach my peers who so desperately need an advocate. We need a medium for voicing our concerns. We need visibility. You have devoted your life to our struggle for Lupus Awareness and I commend you. I would like to do the same. Until the young, black lupus sufferers have a medium and visible spokesperson to address their concerns, they will continue to play an insignificant role in Lupus Awareness. Please allow me to help. I look forward to further discussion with you on this matter. I thank you for your time. SASE enclosed.

Living With Lupus —
A Parent's Message

By Moe Liss, President
Lupus Foundation of New Jersey

I will never forget that phone call — 9 years ago. It was from my daughter Debbie who lived in California. "Daddy" she said, "they just diagnosed what's wrong with me. The doctor said I have systemic lupus erythematosus" — she could hardly pronounce the disease, no less understand what she, at 21 years of age, was about to face for a long time.

The words struck me like an arrow. Systemic lupus something or other. What was it? I never heard of this disease. I felt completely ignorant, helpless, afraid, alone. What did I do or not do to bring this disease on — this disease that neither of us could pronounce or understand. "Debbie" I said, "don't worry, I'll find out all I can about it and get back to you." That's all I could say at the moment — the most important moment in my daughter's life and all her educated, all knowing, loving father could say was I'll get back to you with some answers. What answers — was there a cure — was it life threatening — how much pain will she have to endure — what kind of life will she now lead — how can we as parents help her — should she move back to New Jersey — should we move to California — on and on these questions ran through my head.

All of a sudden I felt great anger gripping my body. Why my beautiful daughter — why her in the early stages of her life — why her who loves life so much and has so much to live for. Why have you done this to her? The you I still cannot figure out.

How did a loving father cope these past 9 years? How do all our parents, spouses, siblings — significant others who have loved ones afflicted with lupus cope? How do you deal with anger, guilt, fear, the so many feelings, mixed up inside of you every day as you see your loved one suffer. When you want to take the pain away and cannot. When you want to say "give it to me, let me suffer with it so you may go on and live a normal life".

I, like many of you, have found some answers and a great deal of support from the Lupus Foundation. In my case, the Lupus Foundation of New Jersey. I first joined for very selfish reasons. I wanted knowledge, information I could pass on to my daughter and to help me understand what this disease was all about. What effect will drugs have on her body? Are there alternate treatments? What about nutrition, diet, exercise, etc., etc., etc.? I asked many, many questions, attended many meetings, spoke with many doctors, got some answers, not enough — there had to be some other way. It was then I decided the best source of information, the best way I as a parent could cope with this disease was to get involved directly with lupus patients. Get to know them, them to know me — what it feels like being a parent. To put to work my skills as a trained 'Behavioral Counselor' to help them and they help me.

I began conducting rap groups, support groups for patients and significant others. I've learned more about the disease, as well as how to cope more effectively as a parent from those sessions than from all the medical lectures I've attended. I found the answers to many questions — the answer that in most cases you, the lupus patient, has more knowledge about the disease and its effect on your body than any physician. That each one of you must become more assertive and forthright concerning the treatment you favor. That the most important aspect of the doctor-patient relationship is, that your doctor be a good listener, as well as someone you can depend on.

In turn I've shared my knowledge concerning the importance of a positive self-concept of feeling good about oneself in coping with lupus. Of how to deal more effectively with stress and the impact of "mind on the body".

We've learned from each other, we laugh, cry, share feelings, touch each other and together me, a parent, and they, the patients, have formed a beautiful bond and friendship. The patient learning how to cope more effectively with lupus, the parent learning from it, deals more effectively with his feelings, as well as being able to better relate to and communicate with his daughter.

In summary, I am calling on all of you out there — All you parents, spouses, significant others — Come and join us, Come get involved — No more feelings of loneliness, No more feelings of helplessness, of guilt.

5

UNDERSTANDING THE CHALLENGES FOR THE LUPUS PATIENT FROM THE PHYSICIAN'S PERSPECTIVE

Reflections...Observations...

In Conversation with Malcolm Rogers, M.D.

So many years after I was diagnosed with lupus, I write and muse about the power of human emotions. Are the feelings of hope and the capacity to love genetic? How can one restore in the young lupus patient the feeling of excitement about life when everything appears devoid of meaning? How can one fight such feelings as sadness and emptiness? How can one help the human spirit to fight adversity and illness? How did Flannery O'Connor write everlasting books and stories during her fight with lupus, while others succumb to despair under similar or lesser adversities? It makes one wonder whether this deserves a deeper exploration by the physicians.

With lupus, one is surrounded by the confusion of the disease. None of it makes sense! Sometimes it feels like madness. How can emotions help the struggle of survival? How can the spirit provide energy to help the body fight its struggle. When you awake, stiff and tired and in pain, and you appear unable to face the day, what sparks the will to fight? There are so many questions I wish to answer for myself and then for others.

And as I always do, when I cannot find answers, I talk with perceptive patients and with physicians. I asked Dr. Malcolm Rogers to give us his thoughts, and this is what he wrote:

I am sure a psychiatrist is not better equipped to answer many of these questions than a philosopher or a theologian. But let me make a few general observations.

First, I would say that most of us in medicine are impressed and often surprised by the capacity of patients to adapt to very difficult circumstances: whether it be to a chronic disease, such as lupus, or to extraordinary procedures, such as organ transplantation, disfiguring surgery, or dialysis. A recent article in the *New England Journal of Medicine* documented the healthy adaptation made by an overwhelming majority of patients with a variety of chronic illnesses. Human beings are very resilient. One sees evidence for this in many extraordinary stories of survival in the face of seemingly overwhelming adversity.

Part of this resilience, of course, derives from our drive for survival which certainly has evolutionary and genetic roots. Part of it also lies in the range of psychological processes available — from fantasy, dissociation, denial, strength of attachment, i.e., the capacity to live, and the capacity to intellectualize. These are all derived from a highly developed central nervous system.

No doubt there are some genetic differences among people in many of these capacities, and probably even greater differences based on learning and experience. Yet all are psychological resources potentially available to the average human being. Patients who start from a point of reasonably positive self-esteem and a network of good friends and caring family are more likely to deal with the challenge effectively. A strong individual identity also helps, as does past experience in coping with adversity. Nothing strengthens confidence as much as experience in confronting and mastering difficulties. The obverse of this is what some have called learned helplessness, a phenomenon which can be demonstrated experimentally in animals.

How might these responses help the body fight lupus? No one really knows, although it seems intuitively obvious that patients who remain determined to function and enjoy life will have a better outcome than patients who are overwhelmed and defeated. They will probably take better care of themselves and be more energetic about obtaining the best possible treatment from the medical profession.

Beyond that, however, is it possible that such an attitude can alter the underlying disease process? In recent years, a number of investigations have explored the possibility that emotions can affect the functioning of the immune system. In some animal models, stress has been shown to diminish some measures of immunity. In humans, the stress of bereavement has been shown in two studies to diminish cellular immunity. Whether such changes in immunity related to stress and depression are of importance in lupus is uncertain. Many patients with lupus have the impression that emotional stress and mood can affect their exacerbations.

In any event, it is clear that the mind and the body are inseparable, and there is at least a theoretical basis for supposing that emotional well-being might have a beneficial impact on disease activity in lupus.

Can One Cope With Lupus?

By Malcolm P. Rogers, M.D.

Robert Louis Stevenson, a victim of pulmonary tuberculosis, once wrote, "Life is not a matter of holding good cards, but of playing a poor hand well."

What are the "bad cards" dealt in lupus, and what kinds of psychological adjustments are required in coping with the disease? In all cases, the real meaning of the illness results from a complex interaction between personality, age and the life tasks attendant to that stage of life, relationships, the physical characteristics of their environment, and the specific symptoms of lupus encountered. This is not a simple equation.

But to take a case in point, Henrietta Aladjem's book *Lupus — Hope Through Understanding* contains a moving personal account (pp. 53-56). Although Vicki* was younger than most at onset, her experience illustrates many of the common issues faced.

Difficulty in Establishing the Diagnosis

One of the specific difficulties faced by lupus patients is the relative obscurity of the illness and hence the difficulty in arriving at a diagnosis. While more education and awareness of the illness may be changing this pattern, there nevertheless has commonly been a long history of frustration in obtaining the proper diagnosis. In many cases, the history of such unhappy encounters with doctors has undermined the patient's confidence in the medical community. For example, one patient reported, "I knew I was ill, but I could get no one, it was never anybody's department. That would be my prime complaint; that if you go to a gynecologist, but you have no problems of that sort, forget about saying, 'I feel horrible. I'm ill.' It's not their department. I went to at least eight doctors with weakness and fatigue before I could even get anyone to listen. I had all the classic symptoms. I could now diagnose it on the phone. Finally, I did get into the hands of a doctor who stuck with it. He did say, 'I'm *going to stick with it* until I find out what's the matter with this lady.' If I hadn't had that good fortune, I don't think they would have found it yet."

Such reports are commonplace in medicine, but they are more likely with a disease which involves many different organ systems and hence many different specialists. As in many syndromes, unless the physician is thinking in terms of the overall picture, the diagnosis may be missed. Another patient said, "I was sick for quite a while and the first doctor that I saw just wasn't helping me. His final conclusion was that I needed psychiatric help. In the meantime, I'm getting worse." Eventually, she found a specialist who made the diagnosis.

For many patients, the perceived injustice of an early recommendation for psychiatric treatment may create wariness about later, more appropriate recommendations. The physician treating a patient with lupus will benefit by knowing about the patient's earlier treatment experience and by being sensitive to that.

Another major issue is loss of *independence*. Vicki described the regression back into the family fold, the passivity, and the loss of initiative.

When we interviewed a number of patients with lupus, two thirds of them listed loss of independence as the "biggest problem" presented by the illness. One of them described a particular example.

"I have to depend on people to help me on things I can't do; my daughter, for instance, if she wants to go out, say in the pool or something, I can't sit with her. I have to depend on my father and husband to do these things. Or if she goes to the beach he has to take her . . . when I first got my daughter, I couldn't take her out for walks during the day. So my neighbor's daughter, she played with her a lot . . ."

In this instance she is, of course, referring to the restriction imposed by exposure to the sun. Roughly one third to one half of patients with lupus have photosensitivity.

Other symptoms, such as fatigue and joint pains, also frequently interfere with function, hence with leisure situations, with work and/or relationships. About half of the patients we interviewed described significant alterations in relationships with family and friends (within the past year), especially spouses (an increased frequency of arguments and sexual problems was described). There were also changes in work and financial status and in other social activities.

Many of these same issues are also experienced by patients with another chronic illness, such as rheumatoid arthritis; but in contrast to that illness, lupus raises another unique concern — namely, *fear of death* and the potentially life-threatening nature of the illness. One articulate young woman described it this way:

"I wasn't dying of lupus but nevertheless I felt I was. It was a constant preoccupation to me and it has never really quite left me. I don't think a day goes by that I don't think in some terms about dying. Although by now I realize I'm not rationally afraid, that I'm popping off at any minute, I think it forever destroyed the sense of unreality it has for most people. For me, it became very real and very concrete at an early age and I've been fussing with it ever since."

The reality, of course, is that the prognosis in this disease has improved dramatically, with many if not most patients having a normal life span as a result of earlier recognition and vigorous treatment; nevertheless, the psychological issue often arises.

Another major issue is that of change in *appearance* and therefore of *self-image,* perhaps especially significant in young women.

Vicki described the rash and also the "moon face" sometimes associated with steroids. She retreated from the world for a time.

There is also the opposite problem with lupus, namely, that it may be a hidden illness with fatigue or simply not feeling well; but nothing is visible. That may present a dilemma: to whom do you explain your illness and in how much detail, knowing that the other person may never have heard of the disease? Part of this problem is that there is likely to be a competing wish to appear normal and therefore say nothing or, at least, minimize it, not wishing to have your identity defined by the illness.

CNS Lupus

Another problem more specific to lupus is that the disease may attack the central nervous system in about 20 percent of cases. The symptoms of this involvement range from psychosis (with hallucinations and delusions), to seizures, to more subtle disturbances of mood and condition. In most instances, this brain involvement is not only treatable with steroids, but reversible. But for a time it can impair judgment and emotional equilibrium and be quite scary, especially to the family. Given all the cognitive and emotional fine tuning that's really required in coping with lupus, any threat to the organ which performs that function — namely, the brain — is an added threat, fortunately relatively brief in most cases.

So, these are some of the more common issues for life experience created by lupus, not to mention the uncertainty about its course and, thus, uncertainty for future planning, the effect of pregnancy, the effect on family, the potential for social isolation, and so forth.

So, I have sketched out some of the more common concerns patients with lupus have expressed. How do they adapt?

Relationship with Doctor

An essential ingredient, I am convinced, is a positive relationship with the doctor. First, one needs to feel, family as much as patients, that the doctor knows this disease well and can provide optimal medical management. That is a lot, but not sufficient. Most patients I have spoken to also expect the doctor to be interested in the ways in which the disease has affected their lives, the very issue which I have touched on. For the patient, the biological details are secondary. The main issue is — what does all of this mean for my life? My view is that optimal medical management must include these kinds of considerations.

Take the issue of rest as an example. That may be what the joints need at a particular point, but the psyche may need to continue to work. Balancing out competing needs like this is the art of medicine.

What if you don't feel this kind of relationship with your doctor? Reflect on it. Ask yourself whether you've tried to communicate as well as *you* can; if there are conflicts or disappointments, have you tried to air them? Is the doctor the recipient of anger or disappointment because he or she can't cure the disease and has come to symbolize the failings of a parent or a spouse? So my advice, really, when the relationship is not working, is to examine why. Try to correct it; and if you can't, find someone with whom you can work.

Another useful approach is seeking information. Knowing the limits of what's known often helps. You can't expect your doctor to tell you what *no one* knows, after all. Generally, greater knowledge of the illness and side effects of various treatments will enable the patient to interpret symptoms and be an effective ally in fighting the disease with the doctor. Greater knowledge of current research advances may inspire hope, which is also an essential ingredient in coping. This is clearly one of the more important functions of the Lupus Foundation.

Eventually, I think many, if not most, patients develop what I would call a positive attitude, characterized by hope and a heightening of appreciation for the capacities that remain. For example, the initial fear of death may be replaced by a gratitude for life, or a more intense enjoyment of good health, or nature, or new relationships.

In the face of uncertainties for the future, concrete day-to-day goals are set and more contingency planning is required. If appearance has changed, other character strengths may become more highly valued. If some activities are given up, new ones assume greater meaning.

One patient expressed it this way:

"You wonder what side of the fence you're standing on. Are you on the outside looking in at yourself, thinking — what a mess — can't do this — can't do that — poor me? Or are you on the inside looking out at the world, thinking — God, it's a beautiful day today. I may not be able to go sit in the sun, but it sure looks good and look how happy my children and grandchildren are — running around having a great time. If I had no eyes, I couldn't *see* the smile on their faces."

Whenever I've asked patients how they cope, they always mention the support of their families and friends, in addition to the importance of a positive mental outlook.

I suppose the most important prescriptions are to communicate as openly as possible within the family so that both the patient and concerned family members don't totally neglect their personal needs in the interest of the other.

---

*Vicki Croke is a typesetting editor of the *Boston Globe* and is on the advisory board of *Lupus News*.

Can Doctors Distinguish Between Neurosis and Lupus Itself?

By Malcolm P. Rogers, M.D.

Patients have stressed that physicians often cannot distinguish between neurosis and the disease itself. Why is this such a confusing problem with lupus, patients wonder? The reason derives from a combination of factors — the frequent lag time in diagnosis, the intense emotions triggered by the disease, and the potential for direct involvement of the brain through inflammation.

The fact that lupus involves symptoms and signs in many different parts of the body, frequently at different periods of time, makes it difficult to diagnose. Many of its symptoms, such as fatigue and aches and pains, are not specific. Some patients will have been ill for a prolonged period of time, during which "not much physically wrong with them" will have been found. Suspicions about whether their illness might be "psychologic" may well have arisen and, as a matter of fact, need to be considered as part of the differential diagnosis when physical symptoms seem inconsistent or "don't add up." Sensitive exploration of such a possibility is usually accepted by patients. However, feelings of anger, mistrust, and self-doubt may develop during this early phase of diagnostic confusion and can have residual effects on later encounters with doctors. Occasionally, lupus patients may be perceived as "neurotic" by doctors for these reasons. After all, "neurotic" basically implies that one's emotional responses and perception are of exaggerated intensity.

A psychiatrist would approach this kind of a question by trying to determine the person's usual mental state and personality and then reconstructing when and how it changed. This baseline personality becomes the normal standard against which change is measured. When was she last "herself" and how is she now different? In the case of lupus, one then needs to listen empathically to the major losses which this illness has created for the person. One should re-evaluate whether the patient's reactions are neurotic or appropriate, given the magnitude of the recent adjustment.

Probably the most important question is whether or not the

behavior and emotional state are adaptive for successful functioning for relationships with friends and family, for work, and for optimal care within the medical community. In essence, the doctor tries to make a very complicated judgment about whether the level of fear, or depression, or anger, or whatever emotional reaction, is part of a constructive coping process or, rather, suggests that the patient is overwhelmed. The perspective of the family is invaluable in this assessment.

Depending on this evaluation, the patient's primary doctor may raise the possibility of psychiatric care to help the patient regain her emotional equilibrium. It is important that the suggestion of psychiatric care not be misperceived as a minimizing of the difficulties of the disease itself or imply that the patient is "crazy" or weak. The point is that the illness requires "working through" many readjustments, and sometimes the intervention of a skilled mental health professional knowledgeable about the disease can be extremely beneficial.

Beyond these factors, there are at least two additional ways in which lupus can affect the patient's mental state. One is by causing inflammation in the brain (lupus cerebritis). The other comes from the tendency of Prednisone (or other corticosteroids) to affect mood. When intellectual capacities, such as memory or attention span, become impaired (with or without other emotional changes), the likelihood of lupus cerebritis increases.

Unfortunately, it is frequently very difficult to document the diagnosis of lupus cerebritis. For obvious reasons, brain biopsies are not performed for this purpose; and the neurological diagnostic procedures generally used — lumbar puncture, CAT scan, EEG, even MRI — are not sensitive enough to always detect lupus cerebritis when it is present. Special psychological tests for memory and attention (referred to as neuropsychological testing) are somewhat more sensitive, but there is a need for a more sensitive neurophysiological test. New approaches to the standard EEG, such as using evoked potentials with computerized analysis of the EEG, or other recent brain imaging innovations, may offer such a possibility.

All in all, sorting out what mental processes may be reactions to the disease as opposed to manifestations of the disease itself, and attempting to gauge their adaptiveness, is a complicated matter for both patient and physician.

What Can Families Do To Help A Member With Lupus

By Malcolm P. Rogers, M.D.

W*hat can families do to help a member with lupus?* That question is frequently asked of the doctor or nurse by various family members. It often reflects a sense of helplessness, anguish, sometimes even guilt over the development of lupus in a family member.

My first response to the family is to have them identify what is most needed by directly asking their daughter, or wife, or whoever the ill family member may be. Expressing love and caring, being available, and trying to respond as specifically as possible to what is most needed by the ill family member and, importantly, not over-responding are the central features of a helpful family response. What is over-responding? Basically, intruding on the privacy or undermining the autonomy of the ill member. That's the short answer to the question.

The long answer is a good deal more complicated, as complicated and diverse as families. Most of us in the field of medicine are acutely aware of the role of families in a patient's illness. We seek the help of families for a variety of reasons: to provide a history of the illness, especially when the patient is a child or is otherwise unable to provide a history; to comfort the patient in the hospital; to monitor the illness; to continue treatments at home which were begun in the hospital or outpatient setting; to provide transportation to and from the hospital when it is needed; and, of course, to provide all of the basic necessities of life, such as food, shelter, and clothing when patients are unable to. Providing for these needs often means that the usual roles within the family may be temporarily or permanently altered. We have only to remind ourselves of a few patients who lacked such family support and for whom the hospital had to assume these various roles to know of the enormous effort required.

In recent years the term "social support system" has become popular within the health profession. It has been difficult to quantitate. However, at the center of it is the patient's perception of sufficient support from family, friends, clubs, churches, and the community at large. (The physician's emotional support is also an important part of this.) Scientific studies have shown that social support tends to cushion the negative effects of stress on a wide variety of illnesses, improving health outcome in many cases. Other studies have shown that rehabilitation from various disabilities, ranging from broken bones to schizophrenia, is enhanced specifically by positive family involvement.

To return to the original question, then, it should be clear that families lend enormous help to a family member with lupus and to their health care providers, even though they are sometimes feeling inadequate in this endeavor.

What is the impact on the family itself? Well, of course, the answer to that depends on which member of the family becomes ill and what roles are disrupted. Given the age and sex distribution in lupus, the most common situation is that the illness arises in a young adult daughter, perhaps either with young children of her own or contemplating having them in the near future. The parents of the patient find it particularly stressful. Several studies, for example, of parents with leukemic children have shown that the stressful nature of their experience is even associated with physiological changes — such as a increase in their adrenal glands' output of steroids.

In lupus and in other diseases in which there is some transmission of a genetic vulnerability, parents may also feel a strong sense of guilt. Sometimes children, in their own anger at being ill, will blame parents, heightening this sense of guilt. On occasion, such a sense of guilt can surface as anger or blaming of someone else, such as the doctor or the nurse. At other times, it may take the form of excessive attention or protection of their daughter. Fortunately, most of the time it generates a more helpful response.

However, it is not at all uncommon for young women with lupus, having recently established independent lives and identities, to feel somewhat threatened or intruded upon by parental attention. Sometimes what the young woman patient needs most is some space or distance from her parents, but their own distress may make it difficult for them to allow it. Families may need to bear their own sense of helplessness without imposing it on their ill daughter, and vice versa.

Young children may have particular difficulty in dealing with illness in their mother. Their stage of cognitive development may prevent any real concept of the illness. If it's not broken, or catching, or tangible, an illness may be beyond the child's intellectual grasp — at least, until adolescence. To the extent that it interferes with the child's life and activities with the ill parent, it will often arouse anger and resentment. These are natural reactions. At the same time, children are very adaptable and do adjust to other limits if evenly and consistently imposed.

One additional stress which may be particularly difficult for families occurs in instances of neuropsychiatric symptoms of lupus. It is hard to deal with illness when it involves changes in mood, personality, and thinking — changes which appear to affect the very essence of the person. It may be difficult but very important to separate the disease from the ill person.

Despite the strains felt within the family, there is no evidence that it becomes dysfunctional or disordered by the impact of the illness. In specific instances in which such a disordered response arises, there usually has been a history of other family problems prior to the illness.

One hears anecdotes about marriages breaking up as a result of lupus. While that has occurred, I am not aware of any evidence that divorce or separation is statistically more likely to happen. In fact, the presence of a serious illness may at times hold a couple together who may have been heading toward a separation, perhaps explaining some of the disruptions which occur "paradoxically" after a return to health. The additional demands on the spouse, plus the interference with sexual activity, can create tension. And the whole issue of children and the medical risks of pregnancy are extremely complicated. But marriages and relationships can be strengthened by such challenges as well.

Ultimately, the outcome depends on the inner resourcefulness of the individuals involved. Psychologists and social scientists have attempted to define the characteristics of this inner strength or "hardiness," as Kobasa has described it.* Commitment, control, and challenge seem to be the key attributes of hardiness, which appears to buffer the impact of stress.

Gail Sheehy, in a recent article, addresses a similar issue in describing personality characteristics of those who have not just survived adversity but have been strengthened in a similar manner.**

*(Kobasa, S.C.; Maddi, S.R.; Kahn, S.; "Hardiness and Health: A Prospective Study," *Journal of Personal Social Psychology,* 42:168-177, 1981).

**("The Victorious Personality," *The New York Times Magazine*, April 20, 1986, p. 24)

Is Sunlight Good
For Depression?

By Malcolm P. Rogers, M.D.

As a lupus patient I have always been strongly advised to avoid any exposure to the sun. But I've heard something recently about the sunlight being good for depression. Can you explain?

The subject of the more mysterious psychological benefit of daylight in depression has been a matter of intense investigation over the past few years.*

Psychiatrists have identified a group of depressed patients whose depression is cyclical, tending to recur in the winter. The hypothesis has been that the reduction in daylight might have a direct physical influence on mood. Investigations have shown that physiological changes in the brain do, in fact, occur as a result of exposure of the retina to light. Seasonal changes in the production of melatonin (a chemical produced in the brain) have been hypothesized as the mechanism of this so-called "winter depression." In early pilot studies conducted at the National Institutes of Mental Health, some patients who are vulnerable to this have benefited from additional exposure to fluorescent light before bedtime or in the early morning.

Recent evidence has further suggested that patients with manic-depressive illness may be supersensitive to the effects of light on their melatonin production.**

The evidence is preliminary, but it does point to the beneficial role of visual exposure to ultraviolet light in regulating mood in a subgroup of depressed patients who are particularly susceptible. It would be unwise for lupus patients to seek more nondiscriminant UV light exposure as a result. However, it is theoretically possible to increase visual exposure while protecting the skin. That raises the issue of how much protection from the sun lupus patients need.

A number of lupus patients have asked me recently how much exposure to the sun they could safely tolerate. Given that only a certain percentage of lupus patients are photosensitive (estimates range from 30-80 percent), how, they wonder, are they to know what their own vulnerability is? How much of a risk should they take? As a psychiatrist, I generally refer these questions back to their rheumatologists or primary care physicians. But it occurred to me that some of these issues might be of general interest in the newsletter.

There is, of course, some factual information about photo-sensitivity which patients need to be aware of although, as so often happens in medicine, that facts are not as complete as one would like. Also, implicit in the question is a more general issue of risk-taking and quality of life in the face of lupus, an issue which arises in many chronic diseases.

First, the basic facts on photosensitivity in lupus: Exposure to ultraviolet (UV) light is associated with skin rashes in exposed areas of the body. It may also lead to exacerbation of other symptoms — such as joint pains, fatigue, or fever — indicative of a more widespread flare-up of disease activity. Sunlight is a principal source of ultraviolet light, but it is important to be aware that a certain amount of ultraviolet light may also come through fog and clouds and be reflected from surfaces on the ground into shaded areas.

There are other sources of UV light as well: some fluorescent lights, ultraviolet lights, sunlamps, photocopy machines, movie or slide projector lights, high-intensity lights in photographic or TV studios, and welders' arcs. The spectrum of UV light can be divided into A, B, or C, depending on the wavelength. Most photosensitive patients are sensitive to the UV-B range (the same range which produces a tan); but some are sensitive to UV-A rays, which can pass through glass.

Aside from avoiding prolonged or intensive exposure, the best protection is the use of high potency sunscreens which block UV light. They are available without prescription. Dr. Elizabeth Cole, a dermatologist at the Newton-Wellesley Hospital, has discussed this issue at length in Chapter 7 of Henrietta Aladjem's *Understanding Lupus*, Charles Scribner's Sons, New York, 1985. She believes that patients with lupus should choose UV blocking agents carefully.

It is beyond the scope of this article to go into specific choices of sunscreens which are available to patients in their areas of the country. However, each carries on the label a rating of its capacity to absorb UV lights, listed as the sun protection factor (SPF): 0, lowest; 15, highest. An SPF rating of 10 or more is essential for lupus patients.

A detailed discussion is contained in a recent review in a

dermatology journal.***

Dr. Cole and other prominent dermatologists strongly recommend that all lupus patients, whether known to be photosensitive or not, should protect themselves daily with sunscreens. More than one application will be necessary, especially if one is out of doors because sweating or swimming will wash the sunscreen off in a short time (within one hour). Therefore, Dr. Cole recommends that the sunscreen be carried all the time and reapplied as needed.

Why UV light exacerbates lupus is not known for sure, but most explanations point to alteration of proteins in the skin cells, such as DNA, which might then serve as antigens triggering antibodies to the self. The reaction of such autoantibodies with other parts of the body is widely believed to be a central disease mechanism in lupus. Inadequately explained by this, however, is why lupus patients are more vulnerable to this process and why a small proportion of the total is particularly photosensitive.

There seems to be no reliable information on the percentage of lupus patients who are photosensitive. Figures vary, and it is important to remember that any given patient may switch from being not photosensitive to becoming photosensitive. Therefore, there can be no guarantee or assurance that exposure to UV light in lupus patients will not be harmful. Thus, there is always a risk, and the safest response is to routinely protect oneself with sunscreens.

If skin lesions do develop, they should be treated promptly by a dermatologist in order to prevent scarring. Steroids both topically applied (to the surface of the lesions) and injected into the lesions can prevent later scarring and disfigurement which can be devastating psychologically.

Beyond giving the facts as they are currently known, it may be that patients' questions need to be explored further or perhaps rephrased. Lupus creates many new uncertainties; that is one of its worst features — for some, the hardest of all to bear. There are no absolute guarantees for remission or protection, just reasonable avoidance of unnecessary risks or, put another way, weighing of relative risks. Uncertainty as a fact of life is augmented for patients with lupus. The management of it needs attention, discussion, and acknowledgement.

What is the downside of avoidance of excessive UV light exposure or sunscreen application? Obviously, it depends on the individual but may include: inconvenience, the constant reminder of illness and limitation, loss of beauty (if the ideal calls for a deep tan), or peer group activities and perhaps some recreational pleasure, or, as mentioned earlier, beneficial effects of sunlight which are only beginning to be understood. These are real losses and can threaten self-esteem.

On the other hand, for most patients, the risks of a flare-up from failing to avoid UV light are much larger. Dr. Cole suggests that sunscreen application be thought of as a kind of insurance, a time-honored approach to risk management. It should also be remembered that excessive UV light has other harmful effects on the skin — such as wrinkling, thickening, or the induction of cancer.

When all is said and done, perhaps the most important point is that, with appropriate attention to the use of sunscreens, patients with lupus need not retreat from engaging in the world outside, from exercise, from friends, work, fresh air, etc., for there would be too high a price to pay for that.

*(Fincher, J., "Notice: Sunlight May Be Necessary for Your Health," *Smithsonian*, p. 71-76, 1985).

**(Levy, A.J.; Nurnberger, J.I., Jr.; Wehr, T.A.; et al.; "Supersensitivity to Light: Possible Marker for Manic-Depressive Illness," *American Journal of Psychiatry*, 142:725-7, 1985).

***(Pathak, M.A.; Fitzpatrick, T.B.; Greiter, Z.J.; and Kraus, E.W.; "Principles of Photoprotection in Sunburn and Suntanning, and Topical and Systemic Photoprotection in Health Disease," *Journal of Dermatology, Surgery, Oncology,* 11:6, June 1985).

Is A Patient's Will To Recover Important?

By Malcolm P. Rogers, M.D.

Patients often ask: Is a patient's will to recover important? If it is lost, what can be done to restore It?

My answer is "yes." A patient's will to recover is important. Although some philosophical treatises have doubted the very existence of will in human action, few experienced clinicians can fail to be impressed with its importance in health and illness. A similar state of disease in two different patients (as far as it can be measured objectively) may lead to total disability in one or to a mild annoyance in another.

Patients also exercise considerable will in their choice of medical help and in their often underestimated capacity to elicit maximum care, or avoidance, as the case may be. In addition, regardless of the treatment prescribed, it is the patient's choice to follow it or not, or to assume an active or passive role with the physician in the pursuit of health. Patients may be the victims of a disease but not helpless victims.

The sudden onset of a disease, such as lupus, does lead to a feeling of helplessness, however. One of the hardest things about this disease which begins so mysteriously within one's body is that it tends to undermine a person's sense of inner control. People are used to controlling their own bodies. Suddenly, fatigue, aches and pains, and skin rashes begin and don't vanish after the expected interval. No matter what the patient does, these symptoms linger in unfamiliar and inexplicable ways. This is, in fact, how people begin to recognize that they may have a disease.

Sometimes, however, before the disease is clearly identified, patients may encounter doubt and disbelief in others about the existence of these symptoms. Sometimes they may encounter such reactions in their doctors. Sometimes, even worse, they may begin to doubt themselves and their own perceptions. It is not surprising, therefore, for patients to lose their will, at least temporarily. Not only have they been betrayed by their own bodies, but their experience has been invalidated.

For most patients, fortunately, this feeling of helplessness will be relatively brief. Time, understanding, support, and a treatment plan will reverse it. Gradually, patients begin to identify what is within their control and what is beyond it and focus their energy on that which they can control.

Uncommonly, the feelings of helplessness and loss of will persist. Their persistence may signal the existence of a serious clinical depression, in which case it will be accompanied by feelings of sadness, hopelessness, mental loss of concentration, global loss of interest and pleasure, and a disturbance of sleep and appetite. Patients caught in the web of this kind of depression need prompt attention from a psychiatrist. Treatment generally consists of specific antidepressant medication and psychotherapy. The psychiatrist must also consider the possibility that lupus involving the brain itself might be responsible for such a mental change.

In the more typical situations, however, a feeling of helplessness will be transient. Expressions of this feeling tend to mobilize caring and support in others, at least for a while. Patients do need help both from the physical demands and from the responsibilities of everyday life. Their energy needs to be diverted temporarily into coping with the disease.

Getting over the initial shock, grieving for the loss of health and the other losses extracted by this illness take time. Patients will call upon inner strengths which have helped them through previous crises. They will gradually learn to accept the reality of the illness and learn more about lupus. They will begin to develop a treatment plan together with their doctor and a personal strategy for dealing with it on a day-to-day or week-to-week basis.

Patients cannot, by an act of will, make their illness disappear; but they can, by an act of will, refuse to let it destroy their spirit.

Excerpted from Henrietta Aladjem's *Understanding Lupus* published by Charles Scribner's Sons and *Lupus News*.

Are Seizures A Manifestation of Lupus?

By Malcolm P. Rogers, M.D.

I have lupus, and I have heard that "seizures" may be a symptom of the disease. How would I know if I'm having seizures? Are they less dangerous than epilepsy?

This is one of the questions that some of my patients ask me. Seizures and epilepsy are two different words for the same thing. The word "epilepsy" does connote, for many people, a more frightening or ominous association than the word "seizures." That may explain the increasing use of the latter instead of the former terminology. It is true that seizures may be a symptom of lupus, probably occurring in around 30 percent of all patients with lupus. It is generally an indication that lupus is affecting the brain, although other causes for the seizures do need to be considered and investigated.

How would you know if you are having seizures? That's a good question and an important one. If you suspect it, you should certainly discuss it with your rheumatologist or whoever is primarily responsible for the care of your illness.

When most people think of seizures, they think of dramatic scenes in which someone suddenly collapses to the floor and shows stiffening and then shaking, twitching movements of the entire body. In most cases, the shaking part lasts only a matter of seconds and may be associated by incontinence or biting of the tongue. It is often preceded by an "aura," a specific and repetitive sensation which becomes a warning that a seizure is about to occur, then a period of unconsciousness for the seizure itself, and a post-seizure recovery phase characterized by lethargy and weakness and sometimes even a temporary paralysis.

No one who witnesses such an event has much difficulty recognizing it as a seizure or, at least, a very significant symptom. It can be frightening, especially if being seen for the first time, and is always disturbing even for trained observers. If it represents a new occurrence or is unusually prolonged, immediate emergency treatment is necessary. The main thing that bystanders can provide is watchful waiting, helping to prevent any serious physical injury from the thrashing about, and comfort and reorientation during the recovery phase. Although the person having the seizure will not remember the actual seizure, he or she will be aware that there has been some spell of unconsciousness unless it occurs during sleep. This kind of seizure is referred to as a "grand mal" seizure.

However, seizures can appear in far more subtle ways, without either loss of consciousness or shaking. There may be a brief alteration in consciousness, perhaps signalled to others by a sudden staring or peculiar posturing. The person having the seizure may be aware of an odd sensation or perception. For example, there may be an odd smell or an odd feeling of motion or an odd abdominal sensation. There may be an altered perception such that a familiar scene looks strange (*jamais vu*), or an unfamiliar scene appears too familiar (*deja vu*). Objects may look too small. There may even be visual or auditory hallucinations. There may be some temporary difficulty in concentrating or processing information.

Whatever the strange experience or perception, it has a sudden onset and comes in the same, stereotyped fashion out of context and beyond the control of the subject. It is recognized as a sudden, brief alteration from the person's usual state and personality. This kind of seizure is termed a partial seizure, and the particular features described are suggestive of a temporal lobe seizure.

All seizures originate from some abnormal electrical discharges in the brain at the site of some injury or scarring. Lupus can produce such a site of injury of irritation, which may be a temporary problem or a recurring one. The diagnosis is made on the basis of a careful history and confirmed by an EEG, or brain wave test, which can record the abnormal discharges occurring in the brain.

Other causes for new onset seizures in adults, such as an infection or a brain tumor, can be ruled out with a spinal tap or a CAT scan. Whatever the cause, anticonvulsant medications, such as dilantin or phenobarbitol or tegretol, can help to prevent the seizures by controlling the sudden abnormal discharges.

I sometimes hesitate to describe such problems in detail. It may cause some patients excessive worry even to identify problems or diseases in themselves which do not exist, much as medical students might overinterpret minor sensations as portending the grave illnesses they are learning about.

On the other hand, informed patients can identify real problems which can benefit from treatment and gain considerable relief from being able to understand and to anticipate. As usual, the task in managing lupus is to pay enough attention while not becoming preoccupied with the disease. It's not easy.

Headaches and
Systemic Lupus

By Malcolm P. Rogers, M.D.

One of the many complicated things about dealing with lupus is that many of the manifestations of the disease occur frequently as part of other, minor, illnesses. For example, fever, fatigue, and muscle aches and pains may all be part of episodic viral syndromes. On the other hand, they may represent manifestations of systemic lupus erythematosus (SLE). Lupus patients are confronted repeatedly with the task of differentiating between the two. Headaches represent another typical symptom of everyday life and minor illnesses; and at the same time, they may represent a significant manifestation of lupus, in particular, central nervous system involvement. So the question I'd like to address here is when and how headache may reflect underlying lupus activity.

There is no accurate data on the incidence of all types of headaches in lupus. While some observers have estimated that the incidence is 5 percent or less, I suspect that the percentage of lupus patients who have various kinds of headaches is considerably higher, perhaps more like 15 or 20 percent. I say that because several studies have indicated that among lupus patients, the incidence of one specific kind of headache, a migrainous-like headache, is approximately 10 percent. It is this migrainous type headache which may be a manifestation of underlying lupus and will, therefore, be the main focus of my discussion. However, before addressing that more specifically, it is worth reviewing the full range of types of headaches and their presumed causes.

The most common types of headaches are divided into five groupings: (1) muscle contraction headache, (2) common migraine, (3) classic migraine, (4) cluster headache, and (5) temporal arteritis. Headaches may also, of course, be manifestations of brief viral illnesses and changing doses of drugs. The hangover headache associated with alcohol withdrawal, for example, is a common one; and withdrawal from other commonly used substances which are not usually thought of as drugs, such as caffeine and nicotine, may also be associated with headaches. A large number of other medications may also be associated with headaches, and it is always worth considering whether the pattern of headaches began in conjunction with the introduction or discontinuation of any medication or drug.

Headaches may originate in a number of different structures around the head and neck. They may begin from sustained muscle contractions around the face and the head. They may originate from inflammation of the lining of the sinuses of the nose and head. They may originate from eye strain, resulting from a spasm of the eye muscles or possibly even inflammation of the iris of the eye. They sometimes originate from pain in the joint of the jaw called the temporal mandibular joint, or they may originate from blood vessels in the head. Finally, headaches can also occasionally result from major changes within the brain itself, such as hemorrhage or tumor.

Muscle contraction headaches are certainly the most common and typically are associated with tension and fatigue related to stress. Pain is usually diffuse and on both sides of the head and may last for days or hours.

The pattern of cluster headaches occurs most commonly in men between the ages of 30 and 50. The term cluster comes from the fact that headaches tend to come and go one or more times a day and may continue in clusters for weeks or months. The pain usually centers around one eye and then spreads to the cheek and forehead and is associated with some reddening and watering of the affected eye and a runny nose.

Headaches associated with temporal arteritis usually begin in the temple area on one side as a transient sensation and gradually become more intense with time. They are caused by inflammation of the artery, usually affecting men and women over the age of 50 and occasionally associated with changes in vision of the same eye.

Migraine has generally been divided into two types, common and classic migraine. Common migraines occur as a throbbing pain on one side or, occasionally, both sides of the head, affecting women more often than men. They may last for hours or days. Classic migraine has similar features but is associated with more specific aura preceding the headache and often associated with nausea. The aura may include a variety of symptoms and, in particular, includes visual symptoms, such as bright lights, lines, patterns, or other distortions. It is the classic pattern of migraine which seems to have a specific association with lupus.

Regardless of the specific pattern, whenever headaches are usually prolonged and unresponsive to the usual pain-relieving medications, they are likely to represent symptoms of lupus itself. In fact, one group of investigators in Toronto, in developing a scale to measure disease activity in lupus, found that such intractable headaches occurred frequently enough to be considered one of the prime symptoms for judging the activity of the disease.

Unlike the more typical pattern of classic migraine, lupus patients with migrainous headaches often do not have an associated family history of migraines; and their headaches typically will have begun in association with the activity of their lupus.

Kenneth Brandt, a rheumatologist at the Indiana University School of Medicine, and Simmons Lessell, an ophthalmologist at Boston University School of Medicine, have been particularly helpful in clarifying the relationship between migrainous phenomenon and lupus. In their original studies, they found an association with changes in the circulation of the back part of the brain where the visual part of the cortex is located. Several of their patients experienced visual hallucinations typical of what have been called "fortification spectres" (jagged lines that resemble an aerial view of ancient fortifications) that occur in classic migraine. Other patients reported flashing white lights in the visual field. One patient's illness began with migrainous headaches preceding several months of all other organ system involvement due to lupus. In several cases, the frequency and severity of the pattern of migrainous headaches in SLE resolved as other features of the disease, including arthritis, pleuritis, and rashes, improved with treatment.

It is interesting that more extensive surveys of patients with classic or common migraine have revealed a variety of common signs and symptoms beginning many hours before the onset of the headache. These symptoms include loss of strength and energy, painful sensitivity to sight and sound, whiteness of the face or head, shivers, irritability, and a variety of intellectual disturbances, including difficulty concentrating, reading, writing, speaking, and blurred vision and nausea.

One wonders whether some of the changes in concentration and thinking reported by lupus patients are symptoms of a migrainous process caused by spasm of the arteries in the brain. There is at least one report, in fact, of fleeting blindness as a manifestation of migraine in patients with lupus which was presumed to be due to spasm of the central retinal artery of the brain. Treatment with nifedipine, an oral calcium channel blocker which dilates the blood vessels, has been successful in relieving the symptom.

In any event, the important point to remember is that when headaches are intractable and not relieved by the usual pain relievers or when they involve specific hallucinations or changes, such as fleeting blindness associated with migrainous phenomenon, they most likely represent a manifestation of the underlying disease process. Treatment with the usual medications for lupus, including steroids, non-steroidal anti-inflammatory medications, and Plaquenil, in addition to the use of drugs like nifedipine, which can dilate the arteries, should be considered.

Could Lupus Affect The Brain?
Could This Be Happening To Me?

By Malcolm P. Rogers, M.D.

I have had lupus for the past six years. Recently, my husband has complained that I don't listen to him. I have been forgetful, but it is hard to manage my responsibilities at home and with the kids since I've had lupus. I have heard about lupus affecting the brain. Could this be happening to me? How would I find out for sure?

It could be, but it may be hard to find out "for sure." Nevertheless, it would be important to look into it further. Systemic lupus erythematosus can involve the nervous system, both the brain and spinal cord, referred to as the central nervous system (CNS), and, in some cases, the peripheral nerves leading to the skin, muscles, and other parts of the body. The latter may sometimes cause numbness or muscle weakness. The CNS is more commonly involved, but probably in only a small percentage of all patients with lupus, perhaps around 20 percent. There is still much to be learned, but the basic problem seems to be a combination of damage to small blood vessels and autoantibodies directed against the brain.

If the kidneys are affected in lupus, routine tests for protein in the urine or creatinine levels in the blood provide very reliable, and relatively simple, diagnostic tests. If further information about the exact nature or extent of kidney damage is necessary, a biopsy may be obtained.

In contrast, the identification of CNS lupus has no comparable simple and reliable screening test, or way of measuring change over time, or definitive biopsy, for obvious reasons.

A wide range of symptoms may indicate the presence of CNS lupus. Psychosis with associated hallucinations or delusions and epileptic seizures and gross disturbances in speech, memory, or movement may leave little doubt that the brain is involved. Occasionally psychosis may be one of the earliest manifestations of the disease, which will not have been diagnosed previously. This points out the need for careful medical evaluation in the diagnosis and treatment of psychiatric disorders. Otherwise, the primary cause of the psychosis may be overlooked.

However, other manifestations of CNS lupus may be more subtle and missed even in patients known to have lupus. Personality change, depression, loss of concentration, mild memory change, or odd spells may indicate CNS lupus. Seizures, instead of being of the readily identifiable "grand mal" variety in which there is total body shaking and loss of consciousness, may be of the "partial and complex" variety. Temporal lobe epilepsy, as an example, is associated with altered, but not loss of, consciousness which might be apparent to others as an odd stare or lapse in attention. Other symptoms might include odd stereotyped movements of the hand or the lips, peculiar smells, strange perceptual experiences, or episodic difficulty in learning.

Thus, when you state in your question that you or those close to you have noticed "forgetfulness" and inattentive listening, you may, indeed, be identifying subtle symptoms of CNS lupus. On the other hand, these symptoms may only reflect increased preoccupation or worry about something; and coping with lupus might certainly account for that, as could any number of issues in everyday life quite unrelated to lupus.

And you may perceive the situation differently. You may feel that you are listening at least as well as, or better than, your husband. You may need to sit down together and talk it out in more detail. If you've done that and don't feel that preoccupation or perhaps mild depression account for the kind of memory or concentration difficulties you are experiencing, then you should talk it over with your doctor.

What can your doctor do to clarify it further?

Well, the clarification process would start with a careful history of these mental changes and a search for associated symptoms, such as the ones outlined here. This would include careful consideration of the role that corticosteroids, like Prednisone or other medications, might be playing. The better the doctor knows you as a person, the better he can judge the significance and meaning of psychological symptoms.

Performance on a variety of cognitive tasks, from housework to job performance outside the home, would be relevant. Your doctor might also do a brief neurological and mental status exam. If he was still concerned, he might refer you to either a neurologist or a psychiatrist or both.

Further testing might include an electroencephalogram (EEG), CAT scan, and detailed neuropsychological testing designed to test memory, attention, and language. In some cases, especially for patients with fever, mental changes, and other signs of lupus activity, a lumbar puncture might be performed. Examination of the cerebrospinal fluid can identify other diagnoses, such as infection in the covering of the brain (meningitis) or mild increases in white blood cells which would suggest CNS lupus.

The problem is that none of these tests is 100 percent sensitive. In fact, their sensitivity is more in the range of 30-50 percent. In other words, 50 percent of patients with CNS lupus will have normal EEG or lumbar puncture results.

Neuropsychological testing is probably somewhat more sensitive to alteration but not necessarily specific to lupus. Clinicians in this field have long agreed that there is a need for a more sensitive test. At the present time, there are a variety of new methods of imaging the brain which offer promise but are not yet routinely used in clinical settings.

In the meantime, patients and physicians both have to tolerate more uncertainty than they would like. Fortunately, most CNS lupus is responsive to treatment (increased corticosteroids) and, in most cases, completely reversible. At times, psychoactive medications, like antidepressants or major tranquilizers, may provide helpful assistance in managing some of these psychiatric syndromes until the CNS lupus activity subsides. Medications used to control seizures may also be critical.

Finally, providing emotional support for the patient and the family is invariably of major importance.

Should You Seek A Second Medical Opinion?

By Malcolm P. Rogers, M.D.

I have lupus and have been seeing my doctor for over a year now. I don't think I'm making enough progress and wonder whether someone else might be able to do more for me. But I worry that my doctor will be upset if I seek another opinion. What should I do?

It is entirely reasonable to seek a second opinion. It is not always necessary, of course; but if you are in doubt about whether to follow a particular treatment, you have every right to review it with another physician. Choosing an appropriate expert in a different institution of clinic usually offers the best independent evaluation. You have every right to reassure yourself that you are following the most beneficial course of therapy. There is no need to hide such a decision from your doctor. In fact, as a common courtesy, you should let your doctor know whom you are planning to see and why. The outside consultant will generally want to see a summary of your medical record anyway. Your own doctor should welcome such outside consultation. Confirmation of his treatment plan by another physician can only strengthen it and make it easier for you to comply with the treatment.

On the other hand, if a well qualified consultant recommends a different course of action, your doctor should welcome that as valuable input. He may disagree, and ultimately you as the patient will have to judge which person or recommendation is the more compelling. In some situations, your doctor may feel that it would not be in your best interest to seek another opinion. And he may be right. The key to it is that he should always be acting in your best interest, not his. If his ego seems wounded, and he is offended or angered by your decision, it is his problem and not yours.

Central Nervous System Lupus

By Judah A. Denburg, M.D.

Among the many manifestations of lupus, one that has most confounded our attempts at understanding is the involvement of the nervous system. Approximately one half of all lupus patients at some point or other during the course of their illness will develop an overt neurological or psychiatric problem for which no other cause apart from the lupus itself can be found. Problems include seizures (fits), strokes, numbness in one area of the body or another, hallucinations or other bizarre thinking, and movement disturbances (for example, Parkinson-like features).

Studies have shown that involvement of the nervous system is closely related to the severity of the lupus and in some studies is connected with a higher mortality rate overall in lupus patients. The problem is deciding when any of these events is due to a cause apart from lupus and when it is the lupus itself which is the cause.

A second problem is distinguishing, among the many manifestations the nervous system can offer, including bizarre behavior and other non-specific signs, such as headaches, mood swings, irritability and difficulty in getting along with one's spouse, how much the lupus has actually initiated and how much the person is reacting to having a chronic disease, such as lupus. For a long time, doctors have noted, along with their lupus patients, that there were many things in day-to-day life that led to patients' having difficulty coping, which were difficult to explain and passed off as lupus patients' just not handling their disease properly. We now know that it is not so simple as that.

The problem is difficult to resolve, since we don't have one specific diagnostic test (so-called gold standard) for nervous system involvement in lupus. There are many different proposed diagnostic tests and many different classification schemes for the various manifestations in the nervous system; and there is no consensus, at least until now, on this issue. The main way of diagnosing nervous system involvement is by history. The clear description of a problem such as a seizure in a lupus patient for which there is no other obvious cause interpreted as good evidence for CNS lupus.

Difficulties further arise when the patient is on corticosteroids, which itself can cause manifestations such as bizarre behavior; and thus the doctor is left with the dilemma of deciding whether to increase or decrease the steroids to see what will happen. Usually the steroids are not the culprit, and its seems as though the lupus itself is somehow responsible for the nervous system manifestation. Various types of X-rays, electrical tests of the brain (EEG), or tests of the blood for autoantibodies until recently have not been able to diagnose this problem with any accuracy.

We therefore have begun to systematically study the function of the nervous system in lupus patients, whether or not they have had clinical problems with the nervous system. The approach we have taken includes a systematic clinical classification of the problems that lupus patients encounter, noting every major or minor problem and deciding arbitrarily whether these will or will not be given the weight of a full-blown flareup in the nervous system. The results of this clinical approach have then been related to results of painstaking, piece by piece investigation of the thinking and other intellectual functions of the brain as measured through psychological tests administered over two to three hours to every patient we have seen.

After having studied approximately 150 lupus patients, with only one exclusion over the past seven years, we have found that many lupus patients have had bona fide problems in their thinking skills and sometimes in their attention, concentration, ability to do designs or recall words or remember sequences or in the emotional spheres and that these problems cannot be accounted for by just being ill, since other ill patients with other diseases do not appear to have these problems.

Many patients whom a clinician would not cite as having a neurological or psychiatric problem nonetheless have deficits on our psychological tests, and this is whether or not we have classified them clinically as having nervous system lupus. We thus have measures of brain function that have not until now been available and mark either unnoticed (subclinical) or early involvement of the nervous system.

It is not the distress that lupus patients have over their disease that causes most of these problems. Moreover, benefit could arise to lupus patients if we diagnose their problems early and plan coping or other remedial strategies to deal with their problem whether alone or together with their spouse. Assurances can be given as to the gravity of the problem or not, and the problems can be more accurately monitored in response to therapy.

We have discussed the psychological approaches we have taken with a number of colleagues, and quite a few are intending in one way or another to look at this issue more carefully in their lupus patients. Others have used these types of approaches in patients with a related condition (Sjögren's syndrome) and have also uncovered a number of problems which up to now have not been discovered clearly.

Since we don't know how the lupus may cause nervous system involvement, another approach by many investigators and ourselves has been to look for a diagnostic test based on what we think lupus does to involve the nervous system. Again, here there is no gold standard; but a number of possibilities have been proposed: vasculitis or inflammation of the blood vessels of the brain which leads to some of the manifestations, or antibodies to the nerve cells themselves which causes them not to function properly, at least, in some patients. Two types of antibodies, at least, have been proposed, some of which are directed against the nerve cells and some of which may be directed against blood vessels or blood components to cause clotting. It is not clear even to the present time which of these mechanisms is the correct one. Chances are that different lupus patients have different problems, but all could lead to the same manifestations.

We have been investigating antibodies against nerve cells based on observations many years ago now by Bluestein and his colleagues that antibodies to white blood cells (lymphocytes) in lupus patients actually can also attack the brain. It was found by these and other investigators that these white cell/brain antibodies may be found in the blood or in the cerebrospinal fluid (i.e., the fluid that bathes the brain) more often in patients who develop nervous system problems than in those who do not.

However, since everybody was using a different definition of nervous system lupus, some studies showed clear-cut relationships while others did not and confusion arose. We therefore began to measure these white blood cell/brain antibodies in our lupus patients who had been well characterized with regard to their psychological and thinking functions.

We have found, quite amazingly, that the antibodies to white blood cells or to brain tissue are found in about one quarter of all lupus patients and more often than not in those patients with problems in their nervous system as defined by our psychological tests ("cognitively impaired" patients). This means that, at least, in some patients the cognitive (thinking) problems and other nervous system difficulties, including "soft" neurological or psychiatric signs, such as headaches and mood swings, may be due to the action of antibodies circulating in the blood and passing into the brain. Indeed, we have monitored a few patients with these antibodies and found that they existed before manifestations of the nervous system occurred but at a time when the psychological tests were revealing early problems; these problems resolved and the antibodies disappeared when therapies were instituted with high doses of steroids and immunosuppressive drugs.

We have also made another startling observation: patients with antibodies to white blood cells in particular seem to have a very specific type of problem in their brain functioning; that is, they have difficulty with shapes and patterns and memory for these non-verbal skills. This implies that some of the antibodies may be attacking specific parts of the brain. We have had the opportunity of doing a very special type of brain scan, called PET scan, on some of these patients and have discovered that we can restore function to some parts of the brain, as measured also by our psychological tests, by giving more steroids or immunosuppressant drugs.

Finally, we are looking at what antigens exist on nerve cells against which the antibodies in lupus blood or spinal fluid react. We have found that there is at least one very characteristic antigen on nerve cells with which only lupus blood samples react, and were busily searching for where in the brain this antigen might be and how it might relate to the problems that some patients have.

Other groups have looked at other antigens and are beginning to define either blood component antigens or antigens within the cell which may relate to specific problems in the nervous system lupus. Thus, the future holds great promise in the understanding and, therefore, the treatment of the so prevalent nervous system manifestations in lupus.

In the next few years, we hope that groups of investigators will get together and decide upon a classification scheme for nervous system lupus and, as well, apply some of the basic laboratory and newer radiological techniques to the unravelling of the mysteries of the brain and the nervous system in lupus. It is only in this way that we will be able to practically help patients with lupus who so often have these problems.

Depression In Lupus

By Howard S. Shapiro, M.D.

Lupus patients often ask, "What degree of depression is 'normal,' and when should the patient seek professional help?" This question reflects an awareness that "depression" occurs frequently in the course of lupus and that there is often an uncertainty as to whether or not it is "to be expected" because of the stresses, strains, continuous adjustments, and frequent sacrifices imposed by the illness. The patient is often well aware that states of depression may be induced by the lupus itself, by various medications used to treat lupus, and by various factors and forces in a patient's life that are unrelated to lupus.

Depression can be understood as a natural, although unpleasant, experience which can vary in intensity, duration, and the degree that it is tolerated by the patient, but most importantly by the degree to which it interferes with the patient's ability to function and maintain a reasonable sense of well being. Therapeutic assistance or intervention is indicated when the degree and duration of the depression is disruptive to the patient's sense of well being and interferes with the patient's overall functioning and adjustment.

The medical condition that we refer to as depression is not to be confused with the transitory, everyday experience of a mild mood swing that everyone experiences during a difficult time of life. We all feel depressed from time to time, just as we feel happy, fearful, jealous, or angry.

Although depressive illness is more common in people with chronic medical illness than it is in the general population, not every patient with a chronic illness (e.g., SLE) suffers from clinical depression.

Clinical depression may bring on a variety of physical and psychological symptoms: sadness and gloom, spells of crying (often without provocation), insomnia or restless sleep (or sleeping too much), loss of appetite (or eating too much), uneasiness or anxiety, irritability, feelings of guilt and remorse, lowered self-esteem, inability to concentrate, diminished memory and recall, indecisiveness, lack of interest in things one formerly enjoyed, fatigue, and . . . a variety of physical symptoms, such as headache, palpitation, diminished sexual interest and/or performance, other body aches and pains, indigestion, constipation or diarrhea, etc.

Two of the most common psychological signs of clinical depression are hopelessness and helplessness. People who feel hopeless believe that their distressing symptoms may never get better, whereas people who feel helpless think that they are beyond help, that no one cares enough to help them or could succeed in helping, even if they tried.

Not all depressed people have all of these symptoms. But someone is considered to be clinically depressed if he or she experiences a depressed mood, disturbances in sleep and appetite, and at least one or two related symptoms which persist for several weeks and are severe enough to disrupt normal daily life. Many people who come for treatment have been depressed for a good deal longer than this — some people stay depressed for years, and life seems flat and meaningless. Thoughts of death and deformity often are present and occasionally turn into self-destructive urges.

While there are many symptoms associated with depression, there are seven which indicate the depth and degree of depression. In descending order, they are: sense of failure, loss of social interest, sense of punishment, suicidal thoughts, dissatisfaction, indecision, and crying.

Depressive illness in the medically ill often goes unrecognized because it presents symptoms so similar to those of the underlying medical condition. In SLE, depressive symptoms, such as lethargy, loss of energy and interest, insomnia, pain intensification, diminished libido, etc., can quite naturally be attributed to the lupus condition.

Unfortunately, many patients refuse to acknowledge themselves in a depressed state; in fact, most depressive illness goes unrecognized and untreated until the later stages when the severity becomes unbearable to the patient and/or until the family or physician can no longer ignore it. In fact, several studies indicate that between 30-50 percent of major depressive illness goes undiagnosed in medical settings. Perhaps more disturbing is that many studies indicate that major depressive disorders in the medically ill are undertreated and inadequately treated, even when recognized.

Stress of all sorts has long been known to exacerbate lupus, and the "stress" and suffering of depressive illness is no exception to this. Patients must take some responsibility toward informing their physicians about the stress(es) and stressors in their lives and must also openly and honestly reveal their true emotional conditions.

Physicians who are familiar with their patients' usual moods and personalities, as well as their life styles and situations, are more likely to recognize changes associated with depressive illness. Similarly, patients are more apt to open up about their feelings when they are encouraged to do so by a physician whom they trust and are familiar with. This is especially important with that group of depressed individuals without the subjective complaints of unhappy mood who often deny or "resist" the notions of "emotional distress," substituting in its place various "physical" complaints. Physicians suspect "masked depression" in such patients, especially when they appear with saddened facial expressions, have lost interest in and withdrawn from their usual activities, and are preoccupied with painful somatic complaints.

Failure to recognize and diagnose depression in the medically ill reinforces the acceptance that they have "reason to feel depressed because they are sick" and therefore discourages appropriate help. This error ignores the fact that clinical depression in the physically ill generally responds well to standard psychiatric treatments and that patients treated only for their physical illness will suffer needlessly the effects of current depression. Depression should not be used a synonym for "sadness."

Today, effective treatment is available for depressive illness and usually consists of psychotropic medication, psychotherapy, and, most often, a combination of both. Antidepressant medication is the major class of drugs used. The four categories are tricyclics, newer-generation non-tricyclic antidepressants, MAO inhibitors, and lithium. The effectiveness of these medications may be increased by using them in combination or by the addition of other medications, such as thyroid compounds. Not infrequently, depressed patients are undertreated and/or inadequately treated, reflecting a therapeutic uncertainty and pessimism.

Adequate and aggressive treatment is vigilant and involves the cooperation and participation of the patient. Such treatment may involve blood tests to determine the appropriate dosages of medication, open communication, trial and error, and a large ration of optimistic support in the form of encouragement, patience, availability, and perseverance. Naturally, any underlying organic factors that contribute to the depressive state must be identified and dealt with.

Antidepressant medications are associated with various side effects and may intensify various symptoms associated with SLE (e.g., increase the drying of mucous membranes in Sjogren's Syndrome). When antidepressant medications are effective, there is a dramatic and welcomed improvement in the patient's sense of well-being and overall attitude and adjustment.

Recovery from depression usually is a gradual process. You can't expect dramatic improvements in a few days; however, one begins to see some progress after a few weeks. Even when depression seems to clear quickly, it is not unusual to relapse when the medication is stopped. For this reason, medication should be continued for approximately six months or longer; and dosage should be tapered slowly over a 3- or 4- week period when treatment is discontinued. Patients who are resistant to those treatments mentioned here have several other effective options.

Often in depressive illness there is a general slowing and clouding of mental functions (cognition); and many lupus patients worry over changes in their alertness, attention span, capacity for concentration, orientation, memory and recall, reasoning abilities, and their use of language and calculations. These troublesome and not infrequent disruptions in mental functioning tend to go under-reported to their physicians and are rarely confirmed to be due to any specific structural change. Fortunately, these transient alterations in mental functioning improve as the depressive condition improves.

Psychotherapy can be very helpful in assisting depressed patients to work through and to understand their feelings, their illness, and their relationships and to cope more effectively with stress and their life situations. The patient's benefits are best served when the primary care physician maintains a close relationship with a psychiatrist or psychologist for consultation about, and referral of, depressed patients presenting difficult diagnostic and treatment problems. Such a working relationship maximizes the quality of patient care and provides the most powerful approach to management of depression.

6

DOCTOR PATIENT RELATIONSHIPS

The Patient's Role In Controlling Lupus

In Conversation with Jean-Luc Senécal, M.D., FRCPC

As a physician providing care to systemic lupus erythe-matosus patients, I am convinced that the successful treatment of the disease does not depend solely on the physician or the team of physicians treating a lupus patient. Successful therapy is also dependent on the patient's educa-tion about the disease. Lupus patients must learn to control lupus, rather than be controlled by lupus. I believe that lupus patients, rather than be "invaded" by the disease, can learn to fight back and join in with their physicians to gain control over their illness.

The burden of having to live with SLE is twofold: on the one hand, there is the physical burden imposed by the illness and its potential severity; and on the other hand, there is the in-tense fear that so often accompanies the illness, even in pa-tients who physically are doing well. I think that, through edu-cation, the person afflicted with lupus can learn to counterattack on both fronts. I would like to discuss succes-sively what the patient can do, starting with how he or she can learn to handle better the physical part of the illness.

Our concept of lupus has changed extraordinarily in the past several years, evolving from the concept of lupus as a "crisis intervention disease" to that of a chronic illness. Many years ago, when the outcome of lupus patients was commonly so poor and the mortality high, lupus used to be a disease of catastrophies, of successive crises. Patients would often go from one major physical problem to another, losing more and more ground with each flare. The major therapeutic concern was to get the patient out of the crisis, if at all possible. What happened to the patient in between was thought to be much less important.

With the use of prednisone and because of a better knowledge of lupus, the overall profile of the illness has now dramatically changed. Lupus has become a different illness, often with a general biphasic pattern. The first phase is that of the acute illness or the period of increasingly severe symptoms that ultimately lead to the diagnosis and effective therapy. In the second phase, the lupus patient is no longer acutely ill but is rather chronically ill. Although in this phase lupus patients may experience prolonged remissions, many other patients remain with bothersome symptoms which, although not life-threatening, will interfere with their ability to lead a normal life and require chronic maintenance therapy, often in the form of a low dose of prednisone.

Why is it important for the lupus patient to be aware of this?

Because flares of lupus may still occur in this second phase and, most importantly, because nowadays the lupus patient is in the privileged situation of being able to help the physician in identifying the onset of a flare. How can that be possible? Simply because lupus is often a self-repetitive disease: the symptoms that the disease has caused in the past are often the symptoms that tend to recur.

Today, most lupus patients who experience flares will not do so overnight; rather, they will experience a progressive decrease in their well-being, often over a period of several days, weeks, or months. And since the major complications of lupus are often preceded by milder symptoms, such as increasing fatigue, pain in the joints, increasing hair loss, etc., the patient is in a privileged position to inform the physician about what is going on.

Nobody knows his/her body better than the patient. The one person who is in the better position to *feel* if the disease is flaring is primarily the patient, not the physician.

It is, thus, essential for the patient to be educated as to the symptoms of lupus in order to be able to identify the onset of a flare. For instance, when I have known a patient for some time after the diagnosis of lupus and the disease has been brought under control, I recapitulate the illness with her, focusing her attention on the symptoms that she experienced with the onset of her illness. Often we are able to trace back those symptoms to several months prior to the diagnosis. It may have been a persistent inability to perform normally in daily life, an increasing need for sleep, transient rashes, a feverish feeling, a new type of headache, chest pain, migrating joint pains, a decrease in appetite, or many other symptoms. Note that these are typically symptoms that the physician cannot see. These symptoms may be indicative of recurring disease and are what the patient should be watching for in the chronic phase of the illness. Other signs may occur, such as the recurrence of a butterfly rash, swollen joints, discoid lesions or leg swelling.

Once informed, the physician will examine you carefully and will order tests to check for other evidence of a lupus flare. If indeed lupus is flaring, often a small adjustment in therapy is all that will be necessary. If a lupus flare is uncertain — and false alarms are frequent — your physician will want to see you more frequently in the weeks to come. At any rate, your telling the physician will have made possible the early identification of a possible flare. Action will have been taken, a crisis will have been avoided.

The key to the control of lupus is, thus, to avoid flares, or, at least, to stop them before they progess in speed and severity. Lupus is like a freight train: it is much easier to stop if the brakes are applied before it has gained speed. And the patient often is the first person to perceive the red signal.

I also like to give to my patients a list of general symptoms that may be indicative of the onset of a flare. While lupus is often a self-repetitive disease, as previously stated, and an extraordinarily individual disease (no two persons with lupus have exactly the same symptoms), patients may develop in the course of their illness symptoms that they had not experienced before. Hence, the necessity for them to be informed on their recognition and potential significance.

Another aspect of how lupus patients can influence the physical burden of their illness is through the avoidance of factors susceptible to trigger flares. Lupus is a potentially severe disease. It is often difficult to predict what will be the disease course in an individual patient. It is extraordinary that lupus patients have in their hands some power to keep their disease under control by avoiding specific factors. I know of few other illnesses that offer this opportunity.

Avoiding sun exposure is mandatory and is much less difficult to accept once one becomes aware of the premature skin aging and marked increase in skin cancer that are associated with the current tanning fad in our society. Although I do not have lupus, I myself avoid prolonged sun exposure because I know I will get sunburned. The trouble that patients have to go through when they get a photosensitive rash is such (topical steroids, antimalarial drugs, more frequent check-ups, fear of awakening the internal disease, and — of course — mandatory sun protection) that it is much simpler to avoid sun exposure.

Another concrete way in which lupus patients can control their illness is by avoidance of birth control pills. Estrogen-containing birth control pills have been convincingly shown to be associated with more frequent lupus flares and should be avoided. In addition, many lupus patients have migraine headaches, thrombophlebitis, vasculitic lesions or other vascular problems; and these are all settings in which oral contraceptives are classically avoided.

I would also like to emphasize the importance of not smoking. I think that this has not been sufficiently emphasized among the means that are at the disposition of lupus patients in order to maintain their health. In the past 30 years, the outcome has extraordinarily improved for lupus patients. This has been associated with the use of steroids, among other factors. Now that lupus patients are living much longer, some of them are victims of a long-term complication of steroids, which is premature coronary heart disease or heart attacks. While several other factors, such as hypertension, may contribute to this problem in lupus patients, the association of smoking with coronary heart disease is such that lupus patients should not smoke. I am so convinced of this statement that I stopped smoking myself three years ago, as an investment in my own health.

Another way for the lupus patient to lessen the physical burden of the illness is to look for things or activities that make her or him feel better. One should not feel guilty at doing exercises, eating a favorite food, or by all means avoiding some activities or even some foods. Throughout a lifetime of chronic illness, the lupus patient will always find some things that make him or her feel better; and the patient should feel at ease, not guilty, in indulging.

Conversely, sooner or later the lupus patient may experience a particular activity or perhaps a particular type of food that makes her feel worse. Why not avoid it? Even though there may not be any scientific basis behind this, what is important is how much better or worse it makes you feel. So listen to yourself.

Another important aspect of the physical impact of lupus is composed of those dreaded symptoms that never seem to go away and that persist many months after a flare is over. I am thinking in particular of chronic fatigue, the lack of drive, the inability to do as much as what one could do before. These symptoms are particularly bothersome and are a major feature of lupus as a chronic illness. After the more severe part of a flare is over, these symptoms are often the hardest to combat.

What can be done about them? There is no magic. You have to learn to live with these symptoms and to adapt your activities to a less intense schedule that will take into account this physical limitation.

I often tell my patients that it is easier for me to treat severe symptoms of lupus than to correct the fatigue or, as I call it, "the last 10 to 20 percent of well-being that is missing in order for you to feel perfect." This is a disability resulting from the disease. Modifications in the therapy can be made, such as increasing slightly the dose of prednisone or perhaps introducing an antimalarial drug in order to decrease these symptoms. But in many instances, the patient has to learn to live with this limitation.

Now let's talk about fear, the other dimension of lupus. In my view, this is the second major burden imposed on patients by lupus. I believe that alleviating this fear is thus a way of alleviating a part of lupus. Lupus sufferers will experience the disease for the rest of their lives. Lupus will modify their ability to work, will change their marital and family life, and will also change their social life. The emotions and the physical aspect of many lupus sufferers will change. They will be sad, worried, haunted by thoughts of dying, even if the disease ultimately is not fatal for them. Fear of death, fear of a relapse, fear of the side effects of the therapy, fear of the dreaded fatigue and fear of "what will come next?" are the daily burden of the SLE patients.

Patient Doctor Relationships*

By Peter H. Schur, M.D.

F ew of us have pleasant memories of visits to a physician. Such encounters remind us that we have, or may have, an illness (a negative concept). We may then have difficulty disassociating that negative concept from the positive attitude we would like to have toward the physician, traditionally regarded as a healer. Why do we often consider disease something "bad", rather than accepting it as something that is part of life, like paying taxes? Some consider even a short term disease a punishment for something we did that we conceive of as "bad" or the result of an uncontrollable external cause. Coping with a chronic illness, such as lupus, is so much harder to bear, because the negative feelings about the disease linger on, as can the symptomatic pain and suffering directly associated with the disease. A chronic disease may result in physical scars or deformities, make housekeeping near impossible without help, create difficulty making meals, going shopping, dressing one's self, enjoying sex, having and taking care of children, and keeping a job, and result in a feeling of uncertainty and loss. Often no external feature of the disease is visible, yet kidney disease, anemia, and psychological stresses may limit one's ability to adequately (as perceived) perform normal functions. A sympathetic physician will try and help a patient cope with both physical symptoms and the feelings/ perceptions about the disease. Unburdening one's self of fears and anxieties as symptoms are clarified often results in relief and reassurance as solutions are developed through effective patient/doctor dialogue.

Not the least of a physician's problems is a hypochondriac, someone for whom illness is a way of life, a person with a ferris wheel of complaints, who physician-hops, obsessed with the notion that all the tests and physicians have missed the "real" disease. These individuals are so preoccupied with their disease/health that they may develop the illusion of controlling the uncontrollable with vitamins, jogging, dieting, etc. The chronic complainer loses credibility (the "cry wolf" phenomenon) as false alarms eventually fall on the deaf ears of family, friends, and physicians, who grow uneasy at the notion of missing a real illness. Difficult as it may be, the physician's role is to convince these individuals that: 1) an annual checkup usually suffices in pinpointing major diseases; and 2) an unresolved underlying emotional/psychological problem may be causing the "dis-ease".

Denial is a problem encountered by many physicians. Patients do not like to hear disquieting news, such as you do (or do not) have lupus, that you require a weight-management program, that you should cease smoking, that you should take (or not take) certain medications, that a conclusive diagnosis isn't possible yet, and more tests and/or consultations are recommended. A good physician is telling you what is in your best health interests. What can you do about the negative feelings you have about what is being said? Many patients simply go to another, even many other, physicians, until they find one who tells them what they want to hear. Assuming that one is dealing with a good physician, and most are, try dealing with your feelings about what is said, and do not dismiss the physician with the recommendations. Trust cements good patient/doctor relationships and in the long term will be beneficial in managing a chronic illness.

What is a Patient Doctor Relationship?

A relationship between patient and physician is both a contract and a partnership. It is a contract in the sense that a patient contracts for the services of a physician and agrees to pay (or have an insurance company) pay for the physician's service. The expected services are for the physician to ensure health and to treat disease. A partnership is important because it is imperative for everyone concerned with health to work on maintaining and improving it. That ongoing process means not only dealing with oneself but also working, sharing, and creating a program with a physician for maintaining and developing systems of dealing with disease when necessary.

Why is a Good Patient Doctor Relationship Important?

Your good health depends somewhat on how well you relate to a physician. You deserve a physician's advice on how to stay healthy, when sick how to effectively treat the illness, and how to cope with the feelings you have about your disease. For that advice and treatment to be effective, one needs confidence in a physician based on a mutual sense of trust, which is a result of effective communication. Trust by the patient therefore, is based on having a physician who listens, explains, suggests ways of staying healthy, and treats you when you are ill. In turn, trust by the physician is based upon a patient practicing good health habits (viz. not smoking, eating well, exercising), being open and clear regarding symptoms and concerns, and the patient following the physician's recommendations.

Choosing a Physician

Different patients require different approaches from a physician. Many simply want to be told what to do without any explanations; others want highly detailed explanations; most fall somewhere in between. Most physicians will modify their style to suit a patient's individual needs; happily, most patients are flexible too. However, sometimes it requires several different patient/doctor interviews to find individuals who can work well together.

In choosing a physician one seeks someone who possesses superior knowledge about a particular disease, someone who listens — asks pertinent questions — someone who will provide answers and useful explanations, someone who is pragmatic and demonstrates determination to keep exploring avenues of resolution (especially important when dealing with a chronic illness); someone who is flexible and is willing to consult others when indicated; someone who is cost conscious, but above all someone who cares, offers hope, and inspires confidence and optimism.

A good family physician or internist is usually found through asking neighbors, friends, family, contacting local medical societies, local hospitals, or a local medical school. Inquire as to why the particular physician was recommended; is he/she Board certified (which indicates a degree of particular expertise). Inquire as to whether he/she is on the staff of a highly regarded hospital, and whether he/she is affiliated with a medical school (becoming a faculty member of a medical school is difficult and indicates that the physician is highly regarded by peers).

However, often a specialist is needed for a consultation for problems beyond those that even a capable and respected internist can handle. Specialists can be identified through the AMA directory of medical specialists, through the local medical society, or more easily through the local medical school. Your local Lupus Foundation may also provide such a list.

How to Optimize the Patient Doctor Relationship: Office Visits – The Nuts and Bolts

Utilize time efficiently: Arrive somewhat early if forms have to be completed. If you expect to be late call the office so that another patient can be rescheduled. If you need to cancel call the office as soon as possible. Bring concise notes that track your symptoms, bring copies of pertinent medical records, laboratory test results, and x-rays. Bring a list of medications you are taking, their names (spelled correctly), their doses (how many mg per pill), and the frequency with which you take them. A list of previous medications taken and whether they were effective, were not, or caused side effects, is also useful. A discharge summary from any hospitalization is useful as it is designed to condense relevant material into two pages.

Be prepared to describe your symptoms and how they affect you, how you feel about them, the stresses in your life, family history, life styles (smoking, alcohol, drugs, exercise, dieting and weight), and what you do (job). Bear in mind that your physician will have to spend some of the time allotted to you in scanning the material you've brought before a productive discussion can begin.

Bring along notes for yourself regarding what you want to discuss and what questions you need answered. Remember — there is no such thing as a dumb question. Be sure that before you leave all your questions are answered. Remember that your physician has probably scheduled you for a certain amount of time for your visit. There is some time flexibility, but if your visit is extended, the doctor will be late for the next patient. If you can't cover everything in one visit, schedule another appointment during which you and your doctor can discuss your other concerns and ask whether he/she has a specific "telephone time" for between-visit questions.

Ask your doctor what diagnosis or diagnoses are probable. Don't be afraid to ask for a layman's explanation of what they are, and where you can obtain more information about them (physicians often have pamphlets available that describe different diseases). Ask about the seriousness and prognosis of these diagnoses and how they are best treated — ask about alternative treatments, and possible side effects of each treatment. Most medications are safe — otherwise they would not have been approved by the FDA. However, some side effects may occur, e.g. rashes, constipation/diarrhea, drowsiness. Ask about the potential benefit and risks of medications. If answers are not clear request clarifications. Take notes. Often a physician will write things down for you.

If you are in doubt about a diagnosis or specific treatment feel free to obtain a second opinion. A capable physician will not be offended by this procedure, because he/she is confident of corroboration.

Ask to schedule a followup appointment. Ask how to reach the physician in an emergency as well as who covers on nights, weekends, and vacations.

Potential Problems

The patient's confidence in a physician erodes if his/her poor personal habits (e.g., smokes in the office, is obese, or sloppy) are evident. By extension, an office that is dirty, cluttered, and disorganized exacerbates the problem. On a personal level, patients are skeptical of a physician who does not examine them for a specific complaint, but instead orders tests and conducts a perfunctory examination. Physicians who are patronizing in attitude or terminology do no service to the relationship.

Hospitalization is often an area of confusion and conflict. Some patients actually want to be hospitalized, "to be taken care of," and think that definitive diagnosis can only be achieved in a hospital. They may feel, correctly, that insurance coverage is often more comprehensive for hospitalizations than for office visits. But most people are unaware that admission often requires approval from an administrator. Many others are reluctant to be hospitalized, and to accept how sick they actually are, are afraid of dying alone, and are unwilling to leave the security of home and family, fearing that spouse and/or children cannot manage without them. All of these concerns are important and need to be addressed.

An additional potential problem occurs when a patient requests unwarranted medication (viz, antibiotics for a viral cold, narcotics, tranquilizers, sleeping pills), refuses to diet, exercise, or stop smoking, and persists in demanding more and more detailed information (yet complaining that medical textbooks are too technical). A rare but related problem arises when a patient actually does know more about a subject than the physician. An honest physician will listen, accepting and appreciating the patient's insights. However, when the patient thinks he or she knows more about a particular subject than the physician but really doesn't, dialogue is well nigh impossible and irreconcilable conflict can easily result.

Feelings About Taking Medications

No one likes to take medications, especially for a long time. When I prescribe I do so because based on my experience and that of my colleagues the potential benefit far outweighs the potential risk. Swallowing a pill is a reminder of the disease lurking beneath the surface suppressed by medication. The scenario is potentially psychologically demoralizing. Discuss with your physician the goals for each medication: pain relief, reducing inflammation, relieving anxiety, reducing side effects of other medication, restoring organ function, clearing up a rash, and enabling one to function. A positive attitude, i.e. focusing on the goals that medication will allow you to achieve will help. Take medications as prescribed. Do not stop medications unless advised to do so. Stopping abruptly may cause a flare of lupus or a potentially harmful withdrawal reaction. If you think you have a bad reaction to a medicine, stop taking it and call you physician right away — if you can't reach him/her, go to a local emergency room for help.

What is a Medical History?

I encourage my medical students to read Agatha Christie mysteries as good examples of learning to look, listen, and search for clues, for accurate diagnosis is similar to solving a mystery. Taking a history from a patient is a combination of reading previous medical summaries, listening (sensitively and perceptively), and asking pertinent questions, many of which may appear, but are far from, irrelevant. Explaining the process of differential diagnosis often eliminates resistance to prolonged questioning. My personal experience has always proven that no medical history is complete with just a list of symptoms. It must include a profile of the patient's personal life as well. A history begins with the patient's description of the symptoms and concerns that resulted in seeking help and ends with anticipated goals. Each sentence may evoke a question from the physician. A dialogue begins. Usually the patient begins with a description of somatic problems. Hopefully, and only when feeling comfortable with the physician's attentiveness and encouragement can psychosocial problems (viz. lifestyle, home and job situations, difficulty juggling responsibilities of children/parents) enter the history as stresses which may shed light on the underlying issues causing the patient's physical symptoms.

Why Tests?

Signs and symptoms, no matter how eloquently described, are often insufficient to pinpoint a diagnosis. We must therefore resort to and rely on modern technology and laboratory tests to acquire objective measurements that indicate what is occurring in the body. Testing, always testing. You see a doctor for lupus symptoms and it seems to result in interminable tests. Some lupus doctors only test the patient and do not even take a history, listen to the patient, or even schedule an examination! Why the need for so much testing? Newly developed immunologic tests are so sensitive that they can now help distinguish lupus from other related conditions. In addition, these new tests for lupus often show abnormalities even before a patient develops symptoms. Tests also offer aid in distinguishing symptoms (e.g., a fever, that may represent a lupus flare) from those that are caused by another disease. However, the sensitivity and specificity of these tests do not excuse physicians from meeting their responsibility of dealing with the "whole" patient, and how he/she respond to testing? While occasional blood tests are easily tolerated, repeated ones day after day are debilitating. No one particularly cares to see his/her blood supply fill endless tubes and vials. As a physician, aware that the body manufactures new red blood cells each day, I can reassure my patients that anemia is unlikely to develop. Having to urinate often into a tiny bottle is messy and cumbersome. These are merely the physical discomforts. The emotional ones can be worse. Frequent testing is a reminder of the chronic nature of the disease. Fearing that the tests will reveal depressing news — especially when you are feeling better and thought you had just recovered from a relapse — can be very psychologically stressful. An anxious patient hears selectively what a doctor says — and categorizes it in black and white terms — either good news or bad news. Tests with comforting results bring a sigh of relief, until the anxiety develops for the next round of tests which may be days, weeks, or even months away. Disappointing results may mean even more tests, and perhaps more medications — with its potential side effects and its constant reminder of the problem.

Although x-rays are less painful than blood tests, legitimate concern about the dangers of radiation increases anxiety in patients. Fortunately, the newer machines tend to emit less radiation. When all the aforementioned tests do not yield as much information as a physician requires to reach a diagnosis, a biopsy may be recommended. Organ tissue, when examined microscopically, will often reveal the characteristic tissue and cellular morphology diagnostic of a specific disease. Some biopsies are relatively painless (e.g., punch biopsies of the skin, bone marrow, and pleura). Other biopsies can be somewhat hazardous (e.g., liver, kidney) and are therefore usually only recommended when information anticipated from the biopsy far outweighs the risk of the procedure. Biopsies of other organs (e.g., brain, heart) are done less frequently because of the potential hazard to the patient. Other tests performed to assess various organ functions include blood counts (bone marrow), urinalysis (kidney), blood tests (many organs), EKG (heart), X-ray (many organs), EEG (brain), etc. Procedure and risk/benefit of a biopsy are issues that should be discussed in detail and at length by patient and physician.

Patient's rights include interpretation of test results. To help better understand technical details, physicians should provide literature that can help explain what the test results mean. Patients may ask for a copy of the test results (and/or other medical records); some physicians/hospitals will charge for this duplication service. These fees should be made known to the patient.

Physicians consider themselves both scientists and humanists. To diagnose correctly and treat appropriately they want and need to be objective. They need to be able to see, feel, hear and measure something that can be defined as abnormal. Usually something clearly abnormal can be defined. However, sometimes what a patient perceives as abnormal is not considered as such by a physician. If the imagined is all too real for the patient, that must also be dealt with accordingly. It is therefore important for a physician to believe the patient's reported symptoms. The art of medicine then can be blended with the science of medicine to determine the correct diagnosis and specific treatment, which includes how the patient can best deal with the problem. Kind words, sincerity, and a clear, comprehensible explanation of what is reality will help allay fantasies and fears. If a patient is having a great deal of difficulty dealing with his/her disease and/or its symptoms consultations with a psychologist/psychiatrist and the use of specific medication may be indicated. Both patient and physician should enjoy a mutual respect, set specific goals, and share responsibility for achieving those goals. To that end, the physician should instruct the patient to accurately monitor the course of the disease. Patient and physician should view the illness in a similar manner, and recognize that their relationship will alter as other individuals (family members and/or consultants) become involved and as the nature of the illness itself changes, shifting priorities and requiring flexibility on everyone's part.

You want to be cared for by a physician; that is your legitimate right; but you also have to accept responsibility for taking care of yourself as best you can. Together you can make a great team!

* Acknowledgments
   The author appreciates the material provided by Dr. L. Daltroy and the editorial assistance of Naomi Storm.

The Patient's Physician Relationship

by Everett Newton Rottenberg, M.D., P.C., F.A.C.P.

During the many years that I have practiced rheumatology, I have noticed new and constantly changing roles for each partner in the patient-physician relationship. Today, the patient is the dominant partner and the physician has become relegated to a less authoritative role.

The noun, doctor, is defined as a "teacher, a learned man." The verb doctor is "to do what is suitable and to teach". A patient is defined as "anyone receiving care or treatment". The adjective "patient" has at least five definitions: 1. bearing or enduring pain or trouble without complaining or losing self-control, 2. refusing to be provoked or aggravated by an assault, 3. calmly tolerating delay, confusion or inefficiency, 4. able to wait calmly for something desired, and 5. steady, diligent and persevering. By these definitions we need a doctoring Doctor relating to a patient Patient to form a positive successful merger for best possible results.

The physician brings into his practice his heart, soul, mind and body. He still must accept medicine as his prime goal in life when he accepts the title of Doctor. He must be an ethical, moral, charitable person who is involved with his family and community.

Many years ago, I saw a young girl in consultation who had seizures, was taking dilantin, and had all the classical findings of lupus erythematosus including rash, sun-sensitivity, joint swelling, pericardial and pleural pains, fever, positive LE Cell test, high sedimentation rate, anemia, fatigue. One unusual finding was the presence of hives over her swollen joints on the back of the hands. Three days later, I attended the American Rheumatism Association meeting in Hollywood, Florida, and heard Dr. Lawrence Shulman describe drug-induced lupus from dilantin. After discussing this with Dr. Shulman, I immediately went to the telephone, called the referring neurologist and told him to stop the medication. I informed him that the serious prognosis that we had discussed only a few days before was not likely going to be true.

Everyone would have preferred to be swimming, but I and 1,000 others were listening to this paper.

The patient has many responsibilities to maintain the best mental and physical health possible. He must play an active role in his medical care. He must learn about his chronic disease, relate his fears, frustrations, goals, share in decisions, inform about adverse effects and investigate problem solving methods to achieve his desires goals.

There are many factors that impede progress toward these goals. Five factors to beware of are: **FEAR, FAMILY, FRIENDS, FRAUD** and **FAKERS**. To counteract fear I give the classic answer that the only 100% fatal disease, is **LIFE**, and that lupus is 100% less dangerous than life. Family and friends become problems which are correctable with proper education and good communication. The only cure for fraud is good communication, so that we can catch those who prey on patients with chronic diseases. Fakers are harder to eliminate. These people actually believe what they say. Someone inadvertently does something, takes something, or observes something and attributes a successful chance improvement to one of these accidental occurrences and promotes this.

Five positive factors are: **FAITH, FAMILY, FRIENDS, FOUNDATION** and **FEDERAL AGENCIES**. Faith includes faith in themselves, faith in their physicians, faith in medical science, faith in nature, faith in the future and faith in religion. The family and friends are positive F's too. When they are able to participate in decisions, and to help but not overwhelm the patient with their own fears and problems. Programs such as Significant Others, help mobilize these resources. In addition the non-profit Lupus Foundation is helpful. The last F is Federal Government which provides Medicare, Food and Drug Administration, Social Security and financial help. The National Institute of Rheumatic, Musculoskeletal and Dermatological Disease is now headed by Lawrence Shulman and is doing valuable research.

When physicians and patients communicate, the patients often become the teacher and the doctor becomes the student. Many applicable research studies are resulting in more effective results.

My greatest fear is that the growing financial powers of insurance companies, government agencies and others will control and change this important partnership between patients and doctors. The quality of care may decline without this communication.

In summary, patient-physician relationships require a patient Patient working with a doctoring Doctor in a good active mutual relationship. Success relies on a dedicated physician who is satisfied with his work, and a patient satisfied that he understands his disease, has accepted it, has coped with it and has taken charge of his life by using all of his valuable resources.

7

MORE RESEARCH ON LUPUS

Lupus And Arthritis

By Ronald I. Carr, M.D., Ph.D.

Despite all the individual and collective educational efforts of LFA members, from time to time we still see or hear reference to lupus as a form of arthritis. Should you become aware of such a reference, we would suggest you send the person making it a copy of the following, with a friendly note.

Systemic lupus erythematosus (SLE lupus) is a chronic, potentially serious multisystem inflammatory disease. It can affect almost any organ or tissue, most frequently the skin, kidneys, central nervous system and joints, as will as other parts of the musculoskeletal system. It is an autoimmune disease, and its problems are caused by abnormal reactions of the body's own immune system. It is not a form of arthritis.

One More Time - Lupus Is Not
A Form Of Arthritis...*

By Chester Alper, M.D.

It would be hard to imagine a disease with more varied clinical manifestations — and therefore, signs and symptoms and multiple organ involvement — than lupus. Any single patient may have only mild disease, with few symptoms or signs or many different symptoms and signs all at once, or spread out over many years.

At a given moment, a group of patients in relapse might have totally different signs and symptoms, and nothing in common but the diagnosis of lupus. Since virtually every organ system of the body may be affected in lupus patients, it is clearly unsatisfactory to call lupus a skin disease, or a heart disease, or a lung disease, or a blood disease, even though it is all these and more. Every once in a while someone attempts to do this.

Reference to lupus as a form of arthritis can be particularly misleading since, although many lupus patients have arthritis symptoms of pain and inflammation, this is typically not crippling. In short, arthritis may be one manifestation of lupus among a long and varied list of other symptoms, and organ involvements.

*Excerpted from *UNDERSTANDING LUPUS* (Scribner's Sons, 1985).

Fatigue and the Vexed, Tired Lupus Patient

By Robert S. Schwartz, M.D.

Four years ago, when February's blasts were rattling the bedroom windows, I too, was shaking. But my chills were not of the wintery kind; the fever and drenching sweats convinced me of that. Too sick that night to think about diagnostic possibilities, I waited for the clarifying effect of morning. But even then the reason for my malaise was inapparent. So it was off to the doctor! He didn't see its cause either; he returned me to the rattling windows for another parched night of rigors. By the next morning, it was obvious. As I gazed at the yellow-stained eyes in my mirror, the phone rang.

"Guess what?"

"I know."

"Hepatitis."

"Yeah."

"Bad hepatitis."

"I know." I crawled back for two more weeks.

When February's ice relented, so did the itching of my saffron skin.

March's sleet found me moved from bed to couch to "convalesce." I developed an inexplicable and insatiable desire for eggs — poached eggs. Breakfast: poached eggs; lunch: poached eggs; supper: poached eggs. Then it began. A peculiar weariness set in, usually after the fourth egg. Lassitude to the point of exhaustion. Loss of interest. Fatigue. It certainly couldn't have been the physical act of ingesting only a few eggs. I thought of Newton's second laws, of entropy, of being run down. But I was better, wasn't I? My tests were normal!

I decided to return to work. The mail was piling up. Telephone messages made pink sand dunes on my desk. The first day was finished for me after only two hours. Wilted, I took a taxi home to collapse on the couch, crushed by fatigue. I slept twelve hours a day. By April I could work three, then four, then six hours a day. May brought its tulips, and with them came new energy and that unfairly maligned ambition. I was

95

back. It was over.

It was hard to forget. I thought about my patients and their fatigue. I realized that at last I understood — really understood — what they were trying to tell me about how they felt, about how their lives were changed by whatever it was that defeated their day at 3:00 in the afternoon. And I began to codify the problem so that I could comprehend better. Early morning lassitude, late morning-early afternoon exhaustion, and twilight apathy: the matins, vespers, and angelus of fatigue. Like those canonical hours, each variation on listlessness signified a different motif.

Twilight apathy, it seemed to me, was perfectly normal. After all, I myself had had it for years. It consists of reclining on the sofa with a newspaper, usually around 6:00 or 7:00 in the evening, and within about five minutes falling into a most pleasant languor. The newspaper slips to the floor. Dozing is prominent. The syndrome terminates after 15-20 minutes with "Dinner is ready!" Refreshed, I eat. The only side effect of an excess of this agreeable habit is insomnia: If I oversleep preprandially, a state of postprandial alertness is to be expected.

By contrast, early morning lassitude is not normal — unless one has been up all night. But given six to eight hours of restful nighttime sleep, the alarm bell should bring with it a sense of readiness for the day, at least by the first cup of coffee. Persistent morning fatigue lasting for hours, and sometimes for the entire day, is abnormal. I am not including in this category those conditions with other symptoms that could account for the weariness, such as the morning stiffness of rheumatoid arthritis, or obvious organic disorders that produce weakness of muscles. Nor do I count here the occasional feeling of being "all in" — a normal response to overwork.

What I am discussing is persistent, day-in, day-out lassitude, uncorrected by appropriate rest, relentless despite a normal pattern of sleep, unrelated to one's labor, apparent in the morning and continuing stubbornly throughout most of the day. A patient with this symptom is most likely depressed.

All too often, unfortunately, the suggestion of depression as a cause of this form of fatigue is rejected by the patient, who prefers a real diagnosis — as if "depression" was only a metaphor reinforcing the sense of unworthiness that brought on the symptom in the first place. But depression is a legitimate illness and a treatable one. Anyone can become depressed, even a patient with lupus, a development which demands the most careful evaluation of fatigue in that disease. Here is an example of a recent problem I encountered.

A 30-year-old woman consulted a dermatologist because of a red, scaly rash on her cheeks. The diagnosis of lupus erythematosus of the skin was established by clinical examination and biopsy of the rash. She also complained of marked fatigue, so she was referred for a complete medical evaluation. Careful questioning revealed fatigue of the type I have been discussing. The symptom was severe enough to cause her to leave her job in a law office. Apart from the facial rash, the examination was normal. All laboratory results were normal, including tests for systemic lupus erythematosus and low thyroid function.

More medical and social history was obtained. The patient is a virtual recluse. She has neither friends nor social life. She rarely leaves the house. While in college, a psychological evaluation was done for reasons she was reluctant to disclose. The possibility of depression was raised but firmly rejected. Offers to arrange a second psychological interview were turned down. The physician's appeal to a close relative was ineffective.

The patient continues her secluded life, worn down by her depression, unwilling to accept help. Her fatigue is unrelated to lupus: she has the localized discoid form of the disease, not systemic lupus. Ironically, she was disappointed by the news that she did not have systemic lupus erythematosus — her search for an "acceptable" explanation of her fatigue had come to a dead end. And her physician had failed to help her out of the morass.

Afternoon exhaustion. My own attack of hepatitis vividly revealed to me this form of fatigue. In my case, I felt as if I were swimming against a strong tide, utterly exhausted by an effort that was getting me nowhere. By 2:00 in the afternoon, the most ordinary task defeated me. Working was out of the question.

Very little is know about this peculiar disorder. Thomas Mann described it in detail in his "Magic Mountain," with its brilliant cast of characters taking the cure in an Alpine tuberculosis sanatorium. For all practical purposes, this form of fatigue is virtually always due to a medical illness of the infectious, inflammatory, or neoplastic type. The associated disease may not be a serious one: think of the flu that gets you down for a week. Unlike early morning lassitude, rest can ameliorate this type of fatigue; this is why the patient with fatigue related to a medical disease tends to feel best after a restful night's sleep.

Inflammation is a response the body uses as a defense against invading microbes. The complexity of the inflammatory mechanism results from two factors: the corresponding complexity of the microbial world and the evolutionary legacy we inherited from our animal predecessors whose attempts to protect themselves against a hostile environment went through innumerable trials and errors. In an autoimmune disease like systemic lupus erythematosus, the body musters the very inflammatory mechanisms that it uses as an antimicrobial defense. One result of this is the production by lymphocytes of peptide messengers (small proteins termed lymphokines) which signal other cells to carry out particular functions.

An extremely important lymphokine is Interleukin-1, discovered by Dr. Charles Dinarello and Dr. Sheldon Wolff, of the New England Medical Center and the Tufts University School of Medicine. Interleukin-1, or IL-1, has many different effects on the body. Two of its important activities concern its ability to stimulate certain cells in the brain. Cells in the part of the brain called the hypothalamus respond to IL-1 by causing a rise in the body's temperature: fever. Other brain cells respond to IL-1 by producing yet another peptide that causes sleep. Injection of highly purified IL-1 will put a rabbit to sleep. Another lymphokine, TNF, has the same sleep-inducing property.

Equally interesting is that substances in certain bacteria will themselves induce sleep; so a person infected with, say, tuberculosis bacilli will feel tired for at least two reasons: the body's own sleep-inducing lymphokines and those contained in the microbe itself.

Fever and rest (sleep) are part of the defense against infection. They are imposed on the patient by the body's response to the infection, which includes the production of specific fever-inducing and sleep-inducing peptide messengers. Your mother was right when she told you to go to bed when you had a bad cold! What remains to be shown is that these same mechanisms occur in the patient with active systemic lupus erythematosus — presumably it does, but the actual evidence is lacking. If it is, indeed, correct that IL-1 and TNF are somnolence peptides in lupus, then physicians would have at their disposal an objective means of evaluating and advising the vexed, tired lupus patient.

International Associates

In November of 1990, the Board of Directors of the Lupus Foundation of America voted unanimously to approve the addition of eight new International Associates. The LFA now has fifty-three groups, representing twenty-eight countries: Australia (Riverina) Bulgaria, England (two groups), Germany (Bonn), Poland, Portugal, Romania, South Scotland, Spain, Trinidad and Tobago in West Indies.

The LFA Board enthusiastically agreed that future Lupus Awareness Months should be declared as WORLD WIDE programs. Mrs. Marilyn Sousa, Chairperson of the International Associations told the Board that a Special International Associates brochure is being developed.

Systemic Lupus Erythematosus in Children

In Conversation with Yves Borel, M.D.

Systemic lupus erythematosus strikes children and adults alike, although the natural course of the disease seems to be milder in children. Let us examine the incidence, the mode of onset, and the clinical manifestations of the disease in children and look at the similarities and differences between childhood and adult lupus. He said and continued "not only will we discuss the management and the possible complications of the disease, but we will also consider what it means for a child and his parents to deal with systemic lupus.

But before we consider the child with lupus, let us speak briefly about the prospective mother who has the disease. Is it safe for a woman who has systemic lupus erythematosus to become pregnant? The answer is: it depends on how sick she is. If a woman has mild disease activity, there is practically no risk for either her or her baby. She might deliver prematurely; but in most instances, a healthy, full-term baby is born. In contrast, if she has active disease, which requires large doses of medication, becoming pregnant is not recommended for the woman. Although her systemic lupus might improve during the last months of pregnancy, it will get worse after delivery. Pregnancy might cause relapse. However, it has to be emphasized that there is no risk for the child who is born from a mother with lupus. Although, in certain instances, the child might have the serological hallmarks of the disease in his or her blood, he or she will not get the disease from the mother. Systemic lupus is neither hereditary nor infectious and cannot be transmitted directly from the mother to the child.

The disease is extremely rare before five years of age. There are only a few cases reported in the literature. Before puberty, the incidence is distributed equally between the sexes. In contrast, during the adolescent years, there is a greater preponderance of girls than boys. The sex ratio is about four to five girls to one boy, suggesting that female hormones modulate disease activity. I asked Dr. Borel if lupus is more common in

101

girls than in boys. Dr. Borel explained not only is the incidence in girls greater among blacks than among whites; furthermore, the disease appears also to be more severe in black girls. Thus, both sex and race play a role in the natural course of the disease.

How does the disease begin? In the great majority of cases, the mode of onset is the same in children and adults. They complain of a typical butterfly skin rash on the face, weakness, fever, and joint pain. But in about 20 percent of the cases, the mode of onset is atypical. The first symptoms can be extremely different. For example, weakness may be experienced if anemia or abdominal bleeding are present; cloudy urine may occur if there are white blood cells and albumin in the urine; or signs of a petit mal seizure may occur if there is involvement of the central nervous system. Thus, the mode of onset can reflect blood, kidney, or central nervous system disease. In rare instances, systemic lupus in girls follows juvenile rheumatoid arthritis. Because of these atypical clinical manifestations, it is important to see a specialist who can recognize the disease early.

Perhaps one of the most common questions asked by mothers and pediatricians alike is: I have a 16-year-old girl with a rash on her face and positive antibody to nuclear antigens in her serum. Does she have lupus? A skin rash and a positive antinuclear antibody by themselves are insufficient to make a diagnosis of systemic lupus. One needs at least four criteria, including clinical signs and laboratory tests, to establish the diagnosis. Some of these may include hair loss, albumin in the urine with a low white cell count, and antibody to DNA in the blood. Antinuclear antibody, although quite a sensitive test, is nonspecific. In children it is seen in other diseases, such as juvenile rheumatoid arthritis, mixed connective tissue disease, or scleroderma. In addition, a skin rash is not necessarily a lupus skin rash, particularly if there is no sun sensitivity. Therefore, one has to be careful before making a diagnosis of systemic lupus, since it carries important implications.

If a child has lupus, what happens later in life? I asked "Will he or she have lupus as an adult? Will he or she recover completely, or is he or she going to be sick from time to time?" "It depends on the individual." Dr. Borel answered, "The disease can strike many organs at different times during its course, or the disease may go into remission spontaneously. Is a patient ever "cured" of lupus, or does one only enter remission? This is a difficult question to answer because if one is completely well for one or two years, the disease may still come back again. However, the longer the remission, the better the chance that the disease is "cured". By and large, it seems that children will follow one of two opposite natural courses. Their disease will either remain active after adolescence and the child's life expectancy might and, in most cases, will be shortened; or the disease can enter a permanent remission. These opposite outcomes appear to be determined by a number of factors. Three of them are outstanding: first, whether the disease is systemic with a multi-organ involvement; second, whether the disease involves the central nervous system; and third, whether the disease is manifested by a progressive unremitting kidney disease. Although these three major clinical manifestations are not encouraging, I have to stress that by no means do they necessarily carry a fatal prognosis. Five years after the diagnosis, 95 percent of all children with lupus are alive. It seems that in most instances the disease is somewhat milder in children than it is in adults.

The management of the disease is dictated by the severity of its natural course. If the disease is mildly active with pain and joint swelling and low grade fever, anti-inflammatory agents, such as salycilates (for example, aspirin), might be sufficient. But if the disease is active involving the kidney, heart, or the central nervous system, one might be forced to prescribe cortisone or another steroid-related hormone, such as prednisone. Prednisone, aside from its powerful anti-inflammatory effects, suppresses autoimmunity. If steroids are the preferred drug, it is unfortunate because they have many side effects. One has to emphasize that the side effects are both time and dose dependent. Furthermore, they vary from one patient to another; and many young women can take prednisone for a long period (years) without any major side effects. But for a teenage girl, perhaps one of the most difficult side effects to bear is esthetic. Prednisone can produce weight gain, a so-called "moon face," or red striae on the skin of the abdomen or the upper and lower limbs. I remember one of my teenage patients was a cheerleader. Despite the fact that she had red striae on her legs, she wore skin-colored panty-hose and was still cheerleading. One has to weigh the side effects of prednisone against the benefit of successfully treating the disease.

Steroids remain the drug of choice for controlling disease activity.

Finally, this leads to a discussion of some of the psychological and socioeconomic implications of the disease.

First, I said "what does it mean for a child and his parents to have lupus?" One has to learn to accept the disease and realize that the cause of the disease is still unknown. One of the most difficult things to accept is that the disease is no one's fault. Parents often feel responsible for the illness of their child. One has to convince them that there is absolutely no fault on their part, since the disease is not hereditary. If both parents and patient accept the disease, this is already a great step forward which facilitates communication between parents, doctors, and children. For the parents, there are usually four psychological stages they have to go through (1) guilt, (2) frustration, (3) anger, and finally (4) acceptance. It is only at the last stage that their relationship with their child's illness will be successful.

For the young adult, the disease arrives at a time when many other problems of adolescence have to be faced and solved. The child is experiencing difficulties with personal identity, dependence and sexual awareness, just to mention a few of the problems facing teenagers. Their treatment should reflect an understanding of these issues. For instance, adolescent girls understandably prefer to be examined by a female physician with whom they feel more comfortable.

How the young adult deals with his or her illness varies enormously from one teenager to another. The response also depends largely on how serious the illness is. Parents should encourage their sick child to lead a normal life, to attend school, and to participate in social and physical activities to the fullest extent possible. Children are much more direct and spontaneous than adults. In some instances, to be sick will depress them; but in others, it will help motivate them. Most young adults with lupus are intelligent and perceptive and have an inborn capacity to adjust to what is still an unknown and confusing illness.

Lupus In Children

In Conversation with Daniel Magilavy, M.D.*

The young lupus patient is aware of the transformation of a dream-like world of hope and expectations into a reality of sickness and dread — dread of a chronic life-threatening disease, dread of the side effects of the medication, dread of water retention and disfiguration, dread of suffering, dread of rejection by one's peers, and dread of a life that might not have the dignity and privilege of illusions.

On one of my trips to Washington, D.C., I met with Dr. Daniel Magilavy; I asked him, "What can parents and children with lupus expect on the note of hope for the future of lupus and other rheumatic diseases?" Dr. Magilavy and his colleagues provide care for approximately 450 children in the hospital's Rheumatology Clinic; approximately 300 of those children have juvenile rheumatoid arthritis, approximately 50 have systemic lupus erythematosus, and the remainder have other collagen vascular disorders. Dr. Magilavy explains that these are autoimmune diseases, mysterious conditions in which antibodies derived from the child's own cells, which normally flag foreign cells (such as bacteria) and mark them for destruction, turn against the body's own tissue. He stresses that the results of this intracellular battle are quite devastating, including inflammation and destruction of tissue.

According to Dr. Magilavy, juvenile rheumatoid arthritis affects primarily the synovial tissues of the joints; systemic lupus, by contrast, is a system disease which affects organs throughout the entire body, including the kidneys, liver, lungs and brain. "With proper care," he said, "most children today affected by lupus can lead a fairly normal life."

He stressed that very little is understood about childhood lupus — not only the cause (or causes), but also optimal management. "These children and adolescents," he said, "are often affected with a severe, disfiguring, multi-system disease which often leaves them and their families totally devastated. They often have fears and concerns that they are hesitant to share with the primary physician."

For these reasons the majority of the children with lupus

are treated in a multi-disciplinary Lupus Clinic at Children's Hospital in Washington, D.C. Included in this "team approach" are rheumatologists, nephrologists, adolescent medicine specialists, and, occasionally, dermatologists and cardiologists. "Dysfunction of several organs and organ systems in these children often requires the expertise of several medical specialists.

Children with lupus are often exclusively followed medically by one specialist (e.g., a nephrologist, hematologist, neurologist, or rheumatologist). This can be unfortunate for the child who has several organ systems severely involved. Out of necessity, physicians must occasionally focus exclusively on the child's or adolescent's medical problems. In a patient with rapidly progressive renal or neurologic disease, thrombocytopenia, or pulmonary hemorrhage, for example, there is often little time for the physician to meet the psychological needs of the child. I have, regrettably, witnessed incidences when patients have survived medical emergencies, such as sepsis or pulmonary hemorrhage, only to return home and discontinue their medications or even think of suicide because their emotional needs were not met or even recognized.

Dr. Magilavy stressed that co-workers, therefore, rely heavily on the input of Lupus Clinic nurses and social workers. "They are invaluable resources who play a major role in the comprehensive care program. They often build a very close bonding relationship with the patients. The children and adolescents often confide their fears and concerns only with our nurse or social worker."

This study is done with the help of laboratory animals, the New Zealand Black/White and the MRL mice, inbred strains of mice which spontaneously develop a disease identical to childhood lupus.

*Dr. Magilavy has moved to LaRabida Hospital in Chicago where he is building a lupus clinic of similar structure there.

Can My Eye Irritation Be Related to My Lupus?

by Jeffrey P. Gilbard, M.D.

It is probably not at all evident to most patients that symptoms of ocular irritation can be related to their systemic lupus. Moreover, given the specialized nature of medical training relevant to the eye, this may be an area that is not deeply investigated by the patient's internist or rheumatologist.

Lupus may cause ocular irritations by affecting the tear film of the eye. The normal tear film is composed of three layers. The most superficial layer is composed of oil produced by oil glands in the eyelid called meibomian glands. This layer retards evaporation from the tear film. The majority of the tear film consists of a watery component that is produced by lacrimal gland tissue. The foundation of the tear film is the ocular surface itself, along with mucus that is produced by special goblet cells that lie throughout the conjunctiva.

Patients with lupus may experience chronic ocular irritation from a disease called keratoconjunctivitis sicca (KCS). KCS is an autoimmune inflammatory disease of the lacrimal gland, the gland that produces the watery component of tears; and this disease is commonly associated with systemic autoimmune disease, including lupus. It is unclear just what the exact prevalence of KCS is among lupus patients. KCS is one of several diseases that are referred to as "dry eye" disorders; however, these other dry eye disorders have no association with lupus. Furthermore, there are a variety of other ocular conditions that can cause ocular irritation.

How, then, might you know if you have KCS? Before providing you with a description of the symptoms that are associated with this condition, it is important for me to stress that if you are experiencing chronic ocular irritation, it would be wise for you to seek out a qualified ophthalmologist for a full evaluation and appropriate treatment.

Patients with KCS will note the insidious onset of ocular irritation that becomes worse as the day progresses. The symptoms are chronic and the ocular irritation is commonly described as a sandy-gritty sensation; other patients may note that it is simply harder to keep their eyes open. As the condition advances, symptoms may be present throughout the day; and in more advanced cases, patients may go on to experience a sensitivity to light. The symptoms are most frequently confused with those of meibomitis, an inflammatory condition of the oil-producing meibomian glands of the eyelids, unrelated to lupus, where the symptoms are similar, but worse upon awakening and becoming better as the day goes on. Because meibomitis is such a common disease, and because meibomitis can cause a dry eye disorder, it is not uncommon to see patients who report irritation upon awakening in the morning, then a period of improvement, and finally a return of symptoms late in the day. These patients usually turn out to have meibomitis and KCS simultaneously, or meibomitis with a secondary dry eye disorder.

Patients with KCS tend to have symptoms that are worse as the day progresses because evaporation occurs during the day when the eyes are open, and the rate of tear production by the lacrimal gland is decreased and just can't keep up with normal evaporative losses. Patients with meibomitis have symptoms upon awakening due to the presence of inflammation in the eyelids; as these lie against the cornea continuously during sleep, the symptoms are worse after prolonged lid closure. If there develops sufficient damage to the oil-producing meibomian glands, the oil layer of the tear film becomes defective and tear film evaporative rate increases; and normal rates of tear secretion by the lacrimal gland can no longer keep up with the abnormally high losses from evaporation. These patients will have symptoms late in the day just like those patients with KCS.

Given the complexity of these diseases and the frequent subtlety of the clinical signs, an ophthalmologist will examine the patient's eyes with the help of a specially designed microscope and various dyes. He may also decide to perform special tests. KCS can be alleviated with a variety of artificial tear solutions, but patients should be careful not to use these solutions too frequently. Patients with KCS can often be helped dramatically by a procedure called punctual occlusion. In patients where meibomitis plays a role, a therapeutic trial of low-dose systemic tetracycline may be helpful, along with using hot compresses on the lids.

Systemic lupus erythematosus can cause lacrimal gland changes that are responsible for chronic eye irritation, and there are multiple therapeutic options for the management of the ocular surface disease and symptoms. If you have symptoms such as those mentioned in this article, it would be helpful if you would mention them to your ophthalmologist the next time you see him.

New Hope for the Treatment of Systemic Lupus Erythematosus

By Yves Borel, M.D.

Systemic lupus erythematosus, also known as SLE or lupus, is a serious, debilitating disorder affecting roughly one-half million Americans with nearly 18,000 new cases reported each year. It is a chronic inflammatory disease caused by a defective immune system that reacts against the body's own cells (autoimmunity). The affliction occurs primarily in women and can be fatal. Presently, there is no specific treatment for patients with SLE.

For a number of years, immunosuppressive drugs have been used to combat autoimmune diseases. Unfortunately, the drugs are nonspecific. They suppress the entire immune system leaving the body open to infectious disease.

At The Center for Blood Research, we are exploring a unique therapeutic approach to deal with the problem of autoimmunity in SLE. The concept begins with the body's immune system. In healthy individuals, a powerful process called immunologic tolerance keeps naturally occurring autoantibodies in check. Autoantibodies are antibodies that attack tissues originating from the same body. In autoimmune diseases such as systemic lupus erythematosus, immunologic tolerance is lost, and the body's immune system begins to destroy the very cells it was designed to protect.

In recent years it has become clear that an exciting new approach to induce immunologic tolerance to self is possible without compromising the rest of the immune system. This is the basis for our research. Our long-term goal is to develop a specific treatment for SLE patients.

Inducing immunologic tolerance in autoimmune diseases begins with the isolation of the antigen causing the tissue damage. An antigen is a substance known to cause the formation of antibodies.

In SLE patients, DNA, the substance that controls heredity within their cells, is not recognized as self by the immune system. It is instead identified as an antigen and autoantibodies are produced in preparation for combat.

The autoantibodies then bond with the DNA to create immune complexes which are deposited in the small vessels of many organs. These deposits are the primary cause of tissue damage in SLE patients.

Immunologic tolerance in SLE cases has been induced both in live animals and in human tissue samples by transforming DNA into a substance, called a tolerogen, which is recognized by the immune system as self. Tolerogens are constructed by chemically linking DNA fragments to specific protein molecules already recognized by the body as self. The most effective carrier is gamma globulin, a concentrate of the immune antibodies present in normal human plasma.

These conjugates (DNA fragments linked to gamma globulin) suppress the provoking antibodies to DNA, enabling the immune system to function normally without suppression of other antibodies needed to protect against viruses and bacteria.

Testing the concept of immunologic tolerance in mice genetically prone to develop systemic lupus erythematosus, has been encouraging. Inoculating these mice with tolerogens (DNA fragments linked to gamma globulin) has resulted in a reduced level of anti-DNA antibodies. By reducing these immune complexes within the body, tissue damage is decreased and survival rates rise.

These same tests have been done on human tissues (in vitro) with similar, positive results.

The years ahead look promising for the indication of tolerance to both monospecific and polyspecific antigen diseases where one or several antigens are involved in tissue damage. By combining the unique properties of the gamma globulin protein carrier molecules to a number of antigens responsible for autoimmunity, it should be possible to develop a simple but powerful new therapeutic tool to correct the defective immune mechanism responsible for a variety of autoimmune diseases including: pemphigus, myasthenia gravis, experimental allergic encephalomyelitis and SLE.

Drug-Induced Lupus May Hold a Key to Understanding the Causes of SLE

By Luis Fernandez-Herlihy, M.D.

Certain drugs can produce lupus-like symptoms and abnormal blood test suggesting lupus in persons who do not have systemic lupus erythematosus (SLE). In the past 30 years, it has been found that the drugs listed in Table I are the ones most likely to produce drug-induced lupus erythematosus (DILE).

Table I

Drug	Principal Use
Hydralazine	Hypertension
Procainamide	Heart rhythm irregularity
D-Penicillamine	Rheumatoid arthritis
Isoniazid	Tuberculosis

Also included are certain drugs used in treating epilepsy, overactive thyroid glands, and psychoses.

How symptoms are produced and who is likely to get them are unanswered questions, but there are some interesting clues. When hydralazine and procainamide enter the body, they are transformed, or "acetylated", by an enzyme. In half of the population, this transformation takes place rapidly and these people are said to be "fast acetylators". The rate at which a person acetylates the drug is inherited. Slow acetylators, treated with either hydralazine or procainamide, are more likely to form antinuclear antibodies (ANA) and to develop lupus-like symptoms than are the "fast acetylators", and their symptoms occur sooner.

There are other inherited characteristics which are thought to make a person susceptible to DILE, and there are some differences in population characteristics between SLE and DILE patients. For instance, although Black patients account for about 30 percent of SLE patients, few develop signs of DILE.

The average age at onset of DILE is older than that of SLE, but this could be because older patients are more likely to need these drugs. Men make up only about 10 percent of most series of SLE, but almost 50 percent of DILE patients are men.

Finally, one would expect that half of all patients with SLE would be "slow acetylators" since that is the normal distribution in the population. However, it has been found that the actual proportion is two-thirds, adding weight to the genetic theory of lupus induction or susceptibility. These are theories, but the true mechanisms of DILE or SLE-induction are still unknown.

In a given case, it may be difficult to determine whether a patient has DILE or SLE, but there may be some clues. DILE rarely produces discoid lesions on the skin, nor are the kidney or central nervous system affected. However, joint pains and swelling, pleurisy, pericarditis, fever, and fatigue can occur in both DILE and SLE. Laboratory studies may help to differentiate the two conditions, because antibodies to double-stranded DNA and to "Sm antigen", which are found in SLE, almost never occur in patients with DILE. Some patients with DILE have abnormal lupus blood tests but no symptoms, whereas others have symptoms as well. When the offending drug is stopped, the symptoms usually disappear within days, but the abnormal tests may persist for up to a year.

Very rarely, SLE may begin while one of the drugs is being taken and not subside when the drug is stopped. It is not known if the drug has anything to do with the onset of SLE in these unusual cases. It is important to perform an ANA test before treatment with these drugs, especially with procainamide, hydralazine, and isoniazid in order to know if lupus exists before treatment is started.

What is the treatment of DILE? If the ANA test has become positive, but there are no symptoms, there is no need to stop the drug if its use is necessary. If there are lupus symptoms as well as abnormal blood tests, the drug should be stopped and not used again. A short course of corticosteroid hormones is occasionally necessary in some patients with severe symptoms, such as pericarditis.

Patients with known SLE may use any drug that is indicated since there is no good evidence to suggest that procainamide, hydralazine, or isoniazid are harmful to such patients. However, it is wise for patients with SLE to be cautious in the use of any medicines, including over-the-counter medications, unless there is clear indication for their use.

Drug-induced lupus is an interesting, benign, and curable disease that may hold a key to our understanding of the causes of SLE.

Anti-Phospholipid Antibodies: New Looks at Old Diseases

By Gale A. McCarty, M.D. and Venus Dartez

Janet Ryan, an up-and-coming executive in her 30s had an unexplained blood clot in her leg shortly after the birth of her first child. She had a previous miscarriage, and there was some family history suggesting an autoimmune disease. Janet noticed an intermittent photosensitive rash and complained of joint aches to her internist. Over the years, she developed frequent fatigue and neurological problems, and blood tests began suggesting lupus. Then, Janet suffered a major stroke.

Michael Kelly is an 18 year old man who developed a red lacy rash (livedo reticularis) and had previous heart valve problems and recurrent blood clots in his leg since his early teenage years, but no features of lupus.

For 20 years Susan Beuch, head of a paralegal support firm, has been wondering why she had a stroke and blood clots in her legs at 18. By the time she was 38, Susan had two more strokes, several heart attacks, two miscarriages and needed a heart valve replaced.

The connection among these patients is the presence of a specific autoantibody in their blood which is directed at cell components called phospholipids (anti-phospholipid antibodies, aPL, or synonymously, anti-cardiolipin antibodies).

Since 1983 when Drs. E. Nigel Harris, Assiz Gharavi, Ronald Asherson and Graham RV Hughes in Great Britain first developed a blood test to detect aPL antibodies, there has been a growing awareness of the numerous symptom complexes associated with them. These include: recurrent blockage of arteries (viz. strokes and heart attacks) or veins (viz. thromboses or phlebitis); miscarriages in the second trimester; and severe autoimmune anemia or low blood platelet counts (thrombocytopenia). While recognized first in patients with SLE, it is now known that many individuals with aPL do not have SLE. Their routine antinuclear antibody tests are usually negative. These patients have the primary antiphospholipid antibody syndrome (APS).

Because phospholipids are parts of cells and are components of clotting factors in the blood system, aPL antibodies can cause major damage to cells and blood vessels by promoting blood clot formation.

One detects aPL antibodies by the cardiolipin ELISA test, the activated PTT or the lupus anticoagulant test. Some patients have a false positive syphilis test (viz. VDRL). It is estimated that one in every seven lupus patients has anti-phospholipid antibodies and does not know it. In many of these patients, the aPL are present in a low titer, or are of the IgM class, which may not cause symptoms when they occur alone. Such patients may not need treatment for their aPL (though taking a baby aspirin a day helps prevent blood clots and is often advised). If patients have a stroke, recurrent blood clots, or multiple miscarriages, treatment to decrease antibody production may be considered. Patients who have high levels of the IgG type of aPL seem to be at increased risk for strokes. Preventive treatment should be considered in these patients even if they haven't yet had symptoms. Since the complications associated with these aPL antibodies are often preventable or treatable, early detection is very important for both SLE patients and patients with APS.

Treatment of patients with anti-phospholipid antibodies involves different classes of drugs: aspirin, blood thinners and steroids. Some patients may also need immunosuppressive drugs (viz. azathioprine) in addition to prednisone to decrease antibody production. Patients receiving any of these treatments must be carefully monitored.

Possible Involvement of a Newly Discovered Human Retrovirus in Autoimmunity*

By Robert F. Garry, Ph.D.

In a recent article appearing in *Science* magazine we reported the detection of a previously unknown human retrovirus in cultures of two patients with Sjögren's Syndrome.[1] We named this retrovirus the human intracisternal A-type retroviral particle (HIAP). We have found that many patients with Sjögren's Syndrome and lupus make antibodies that bind to HIAP proteins. This raises the possibility, far from proven, that HIAP might be involved in Sjögren's Syndrome and perhaps in lupus or other autoimmune diseases. As with other discoveries this one raises many questions. The purpose of this article is to clarify what the discovery of a retrovirus with a possible association with autoimmunity means to lupus patients.

What is a retrovirus?

Viruses and retroviruses are parasites which must enter cells to reproduce. Retroviruses differ from other viruses in that they convert their genetic material (which is RNA) into DNA using a retroviral enzyme called reverse transcriptase (Figure 1). This viral DNA copy can *integrate* or become part of the host's own genes (these genes are also DNA). This ability to integrate its genes into the host DNA enables a retrovirus to enter a state of dormancy (also known as latency or persistence). The body cannot completely eliminate a virus in such a dormant state. That is why retrovirus infections may last a lifetime; the retroviral genes become a part of the genetic makeup of the infected person. In integrated form, the retrovirus can either be expressed chronically (thereby slowly inflicting damage) or it may be activated sporadically by factors such as stress or hormones.

A link between autoimmune diseases and retroviruses

An association between retroviruses and human autoimmune diseases has long been suspected. As in many biomedical endeavors our most instructive lessons have come from experimental animals. A retrovirus has been proven to cause chronic arthritis in goats. Another retrovirus has been linked to a version of lupus in mice. Genetically engineered mice expressing a gene of a human retrovirus known as HTLV have recently been shown to develop symptoms resembling Sjögren's Syndrome. Dr. Edward Kuff at the National Cancer Institute has implicated a mouse intracisternal A-type retroviral particle in a form of autoimmune diabetes. Moreover, the worldwide epidemic of a human retrovirus human immunodeficiency virus (HIV) has strengthened the notion that a retrovirus can cause dysfunction of the human immune system. Many symptoms of HIV infection are similar to symptoms of the autoimmune diseases. A few patients infected with HIV develop diseases resembling autoimmune thrombocytopenia, rheumatoid arthritis, lupus or Sjögren's Syndrome. Many HIV-infected persons make low levels of autoantibodies. The late stage of HIV infection results in the Acquired Immune Deficiency Syndrome (AIDS).

We began our studies of a possible retrovirus involvement in autoimmunity with Sjögren's Syndrome. The characteristic symptom of Sjögren's Syndrome is dryness of the mouth and eyes. It was interesting to us that this symptom is also sometimes observed as a manifestation of HIV infection. The dryness in both Sjögren's Syndrome and HIV disease is due to loss of salivary and tear gland function. This is caused by (or at least is accompanied by) infiltration of these glands by lymphocytes, a key cell in the immune system. An additional link between Sjögren's Syndrome and retroviruses is our observation that the immune systems of a significant number (30%) of primary Sjögren's Syndrome patients produce antibodies that react with a major protein of HIV. Similar percentages of lupus, scleroderma, and juvenile rheumatoid arthritis patients also produce retrovirus-reactive serum antibodies. These observations suggested the possibility of a retroviral etiology in these autoimmune diseases. They also suggested the possibility that the retrovirus may be a distant cousin of HIV, but at the same time they indicated conclusively that *HIV or a closer relative of HIV is not involved in autoimmunity.* Importantly, they indicated that some persons with autoimmune diseases may give a false positive result in the tests used to screen donated blood for HIV infection. Persons who repeatedly give *indeterminate* Western blots with rheumatic symptoms and have no risk factors for AIDS are not HIV-infected.

The pathology of early Sjögren's Syndrome is more localized than other autoimmune diseases and is confined mostly to the tear and salivary glands. Later in the course of Sjögren's Syndrome some patients develop rheumatoid arthritis, lupus or other more widespread manifestations. Therefore, we attempted to culture an infectious agent from Sjögren's Syndrome patients at an early stage in their disease. Tissue was collected from the minor salivary glands found in the lips, and homogenates of this tissue were added to cultures of a T-cell line. After several weeks, we were able to detect retrovirus proteins in some of these cultures. This suggests that a retrovirus in the salivary glands had been passed to the cultures and that the cells were now producing a retrovirus.

The newly discovered retrovirus is distinct from HIV and does not cause AIDS

Retroviruses are classified as types A - D according to how they assemble their virus particle and their final structure as determined by electron microscopy (Figure 2). HIV, a subgroup of C-type retroviruses termed lentiviruses, matures at the plasma membrane of infected T-cells, as do retroviruses of types B and D. HIV differs dramatically from HIAP in structure. The HIAP-containing lymphoid cells do not produce viral particles that mature at the plasma membrane like HIV. Instead we observe retroviruses contained within vacuoles inside the cell. The "intracisternal" particles consist of two electron dense concentric rings having a "doughnut-shaped" appearance. This is typical of A-type retroviruses (Figure 2), although prior to our findings human A-type retroviruses were not known to exist. We also have found that the HIAP enzyme reverse transcriptase (that converts the viral RNA into DNA) differs by several important biochemical parameters from the reverse transcriptase of HIV. Furthermore, we used a very specific gene analysis method termed polymerase chain reaction to confirm that HIAP is not simply a variant of HIV.

Our studies also indicate that the HIAP is not contagious like the retrovirus that causes AIDS. One important feature of A-type retroviruses such as HIAP is that they are not infectious by the routes used by other retroviruses such as HIV or by more conventional viruses. We were able to pass HIAP to our cultured cells *only* under the special conditions in the laboratory. In people, the HIAP may be an endogenous retrovirus that is only passed genetically (that is from parent to offspring). Endogenous retroviruses have already been implicated in animal models of lupus by Drs. Arthur Krieg and Alfred Steinberg at the National Institutes of Health. Even if HIAP is shown to have a role in autoimmunity, a variety of genetic, environmental or hormonal factors are also likely to be involved. Thus, not everyone with HIAP will necessarily develop a disease state.

How could a retrovirus induce autoimmune disease?

One means by which a retrovirus might induce autoimmunity is by a process called molecular or antigenic mimicry. Viruses, like other infectious agents and living cells of all organisms, contain proteins, nucleic acids and other compounds that under the right circumstances may be recognized by the human immune system. The immune system is able to discriminate the proteins of most infectious agents as foreign and is able to produce antibodies or immune cells to eliminate the invading entity. Sometimes infectious agents produce proteins that are similar to or mimic host proteins, perhaps as a method of camouflage. People do not usually produce an immune response against their own tissues. However, if the immune system does recognize these host-mimicking proteins on an infectious agent and produces an immune response to them, then the same response might also attack host tissues, a so-called autoimmune response. Other factors no doubt also come into play in determining if a person will actually develop an autoimmune disease, including the influence of genetics, hormones, environment, and perhaps additional infectious agents.

Future plans

The studies discussed here do not provide proof that the agent we have identified is involved in the etiology of Sjögren's Syndrome, lupus or other autoimmune diseases. Nevertheless, the discovery of a human retrovirus associated with autoimmunity is cause for cautious optimism. If we are able to demonstrate a role for this retrovirus in autoimmune disease, this might be a definitive target for therapy. One could envision the development of specific antiretroviral drugs to treat the diseases. It might also be possible to develop vaccines or immunotherapies to prevent expression of the retrovirus.

Many patients have questions regarding recent media reports on retroviruses and autoimmunity. This article is written in the hopes of answering some of these questions.

Figure Legends

Figure 1. Replication of conventional viruses and retroviruses. Most viruses replicate hundreds or thousands of copies of their genes (viral RNA or DNA) which they incorporate directly into progeny viruses. Retroviruses convert their genes which are RNA into DNA using the retrovirus-specified enzyme reverse transcriptase. This viral DNA copy can integrate and become part of the host's own DNA genes. This enables the retrovirus to establish a state of persistence.

Figure 2. Differences in structure and development of different types of retroviruses. Retroviruses are classified into four general types depending on where they assemble in the cell and their final structures. A-type retroviruses assemble inside of the cells and are not contagious. Retrovirus types B - D assemble at the cell surface. B - D type retroviruses are released from the cells, and are thereby contagious.

1. ("Detection of a human intracisternal A-type retroviral particle antigenically related to HIV" Robert F. Garry, Cesar D. Fermin, Darrenn J. Hart, Steve S. Alexander, Lawrence A. Donehower, Hong Luo-Zhang *Science* 250, 1127-1129, 1990)

Figure 1.   Figure 2.

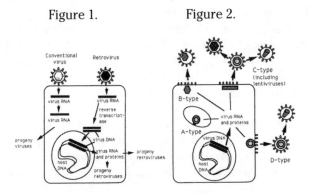

Interpretation of Laboratory Tests

By Peter H. Schur, M.D.

Many tests are done on patients with suspected lupus in order to establish a diagnosis. In patients with systemic lupus erythematosus (SLE), tests are performed to determine which organs are involved, to what extent, and also to determine the degree of activity of the lupus.

Diagnosis

1. *Anti-nuclear antibody tests (ANA, ANF):* This test determines whether a patient has antibodies to the nuclear portion of cells. As a source of nuclei one uses either a cell line (called Hep-2) or micro-thin sections of rat or mouse liver or kidney. The reaction is examined under a microscope. If the reaction is positive, serial dilutions are made of sera. The last dilution of serum still giving a positive reaction is referred to as the titer (e.g., 1/10, 1/40, 1/160, etc.)

Only 14 of 10,000 SLE cases have a negative ANA test.

Thus over 99% of SLE patients have a positive ANA test.

Only 1 of three people with a positive ANA test done with rodent tissue have SLE — the higher the titer the more likely one has SLE.

Only 1 of six people with a positive ANA using Hep-2 cells have SLE — the higher the titer the more likely one has SLE.

Because of variation in technique, results (e.g. titer) may vary from lab to lab — even negative and positive.

2. *Anti-double-stranded DNA antibody (anti-DNA, anti-dsDNA):* This test is performed in different labs by different techniques called radioimmunoassay (RIA, Farr), Crithidia, or enzyme immunoassay (EIA, ELISA). Each lab determines a range of units observed in normals; anything above this range is considered abnormal or positive.

About 75% of patients with SLE have antibodies to dsDNA.

About 95% of patients with antibodies to dsDNA have SLE.

3. *Anti-Sm antibody (Anti-Smith):* Anti-Sm antibodies recognize a unique nuclear RNA-protein complex. This test is per-

formed by either hemagglutination (resulting in a titer), counterimmunoelectrophoresis (usually reported as positive or negative — occasionally as a titer), and most recently by EIA (ELISA) — and reported usually in units.

About 25% of patients with SLE have anti-Sm.

Between 75 and 95% of patients with anti-Sm have SLE.

4. *Anti-RNP (anti-U1-RNP):* Anti-RNP antibodies recognize another unique nuclear RNA-protein complex. This test is performed in a fashion similar to anti-Sm.

About 40% of patients with SLE have anti-RNP.

About 50% of patients with anti-RNP have SLE; others may have MCTD (mixed connective tissue disease), scleroderma, rheumatoid arthritis, Sjögren's syndrome, or related forms of undifferentiated forms of connective tissue disorders.

5. *Anti-Ro (SS-A):* Anti-Ro antibodies recognize another unique nuclear RNA-protein complex. This test is performed by counterimmunoelectrophoresis or EIA.

About 40% of patients with SLE have anti-Ro.

If a patient has anti-Ro one generally considers that the patient has either SLE, Sjögren's syndrome, or photosensitivity.

6. *Anti-La (SS-B):* Anti-La antibodies recognize another unique RNA-protein complex. This test is performed in a manner similar to anti-Ro.

About 30% of SLE patients have anti-La.

If a patient has anti-La one considers SLE or Sjögren's syndrome.

As different labs use different methods for detecting anti-Sm, RNP, Ro and La, results may vary from lab to lab. Furthermore, results of these tests, as well as all others mentioned here, vary over time.

7. *Complement (CH50, C4, C3):* The complement system represents a group of over 20 serum proteins that are activated by reacting with antibodies bound to antigen and then interact to cause inflammation. Thus low levels of complement reflect active disease. The total complement system (CH50) is measured by a hemolytic technique (the release of hemoglobin from specially sensitized sheep red blood cells); C4, and C3 (two of the more important components) are measured by immunodiffusion (reaction of antibody and antigen in agar (a semi-solid medium) — quantitation is determined by the size of a ring; or nephelometry (reaction of antibody and antigen in a fluid — quantitation is determined by optical density). Be-

cause of some variations in technique, each laboratory has established a normal range. A low CH50, C4, or C3 level in conjunction with a positive ANA test is highly suggestive but not diagnostic for SLE.

8. *CBC (Complete Blood Count):* Consisting of a white blood cell count (wbc), hemoglobin (Hgb), hematocrit (Hct) and platelet count is usually performed on an automated machine. The normal range is very well standardized internationally. Low levels of any of these counts in the presence of a positive ANA test are highly suggestive of lupus.

Laboratory Tests for the Assessment of Activity of Lupus

1. ANA: Generally speaking if an ANA titer rises (at least 4 dilutions) it suggests that the lupus may be more active.

2. Anti-DNA: rising titers of anti-DNA are moderately strong indicators that the lupus is becoming more active.

3. Anti-Sm, RNP, Ro, La: there is no evidence that titers (levels) correlate with lupus activity.

4. Complement: Falling (or just low levels) suggest active lupus.

5. CBC: Falling levels of a wbc, Hgb (or Hct), or platelet count suggest active lupus — but other causes (viz drugs, intestinal bleeding) should be excluded. An elevated wbc suggests either infection or taking moderate to high doses of prednisone.

6. Kidney: increasing amounts of protein, rbc, wbc, or a falling GFR reflect worsening kidney function, which may be due to lupus. Often a kidney biopsy needs to be performed to distinguish lupus nephritis from other causes of nephritis.

7. Brain: a worsening MRI or EEG suggests lupus (or other) brain involvement.

Miscellaneous

1. *Anti-cardiolipin antibodies (anti-phospholipid antibodies):* This test is either performed as an EIA or as a modified prothrombin time (a blood coagulation test.) Very high (but not minimally elevated) levels are associated with phlebitis, small strokes, blood vessel occlusions, low platelet counts, and recurrent miscarriages in the 2nd trimester.

Assessing Organ Involvement

1. *Kidney Function Tests*

a). *Urinalysis:* Urine is examined both by dipsticks and microscopically. Normal urine contains no protein, sugar, but may contain up to 5 red blood cells (5 rbc/hpf) or 5 white blood cells (5 wbc/hpf). Presence of protein or more cells suggests inflammation of the kidney, as in lupus nephritis. Absence of urine abnormalities is very strong evidence against the presence of lupus nephritis. The presence of only white blood cells suggests a urinary tract infection.

b). *Serum Creatinine:* Creatinine (a substance in blood) is normally cleared from the blood by the kidney. If there is significant impairment of kidney function, then the serum creatinine is increased.

c). *24 Hour Urine:* One can determine the amount of protein per 24 hours. This fluctuates to some degree. Steady increases of urinary protein means worsening kidney function. One can also determine serum and (24 hour) urine creatinine and calculate a GFR (glomerular filtration rate). This is a sensitive index of kidney function. Normals have values over 100-120.

2. *Brain Involvement*

a). Magnetic resonance imaging (MRI, NMR) is a sensitive nonradioactive technique that often will detect neurological abnormalities in SLE patients.

b). CT scan (CAT scan — computerized tomography) may detect abnormalities in SLE; it has been mostly replaced by the MRI.

c). Brain wave (EEG) — often performed after sleep deprivation or with auditory or visual stimulation. The test is used to detect seizure disorders.

d). Psychological testing (e.g. MMPI): To help distinguish neurological from psychological causes of symptoms.

If all the above are negative, it is highly unlikely that there is lupus brain involvement.

The Antiphospholipid Syndrome

By Daniel J. Wallace, M.D., F.A.C.P., F.A.C.A.
and Allan L. Metzger, M.D.

In the 1940s, it became apparent that many lupus patients had false positive premarital syphilis blood tests. Since none of them had syphilis and no unusual complications were reported, it was considered a laboratory curiosity. In the 1950s, several lupus patients were found to have prolonged blood prothrombin times that seemed to be due to a laboratory artifact and had no association with abnormal bleeding. Known as the lupus anticoagulant, no clinical correlation or significance was attached to this observation. The description of the anticardiolipin antibody by a British group in the early 1980s changed all this. It turns out that about one-third of all lupus patients have antibodies to phospholipids, which make up cell membranes. Some of these were detected by the syphilis serology, some by the blood clotting test, but most by a newly-developed test called the anticardiolipin (or anti-phospholipid) antibody test, since phospholipids were used in the testing procedures. The discovery of certain clinical associations with the presence of these antibodies has resulted in calling this entity the "Antiphospholipid Syndrome" or APL.

Only about one-third of SLE patients with antiphospholipid antibodies ever experience a complication associated with APL. In addition, up to 20% of rheumatoid arthritis patients and 10%-20% with other forms of rheumatic diseases possess these antibodies. Perhaps 1%-2% of the normal population also has anti-phospholipid antibodies, and it has been found in certain infectious diseases. Intense efforts are underway to determine which subgroups are at risk for APL complications, and so far the only truly high risk subset consists of those who have high titers of IgG anticardiolipin antibodies.

The best documented clinical sequelae of APL are: phlebitis with emboli to the lungs, low platelet counts, and recurrent second trimester miscarriages. Other reports have associated APL with avascular necrosis, small strokes, hemolytic anemia, Libman-Sacks endocarditis, and livedo reticulosis. Despite the misnomer "lupus anticoagulant", APL induces clotting as opposed to bleeding. The mechanism by which this occurs is still quite controversial, but no doubt has to do with an interaction between phospholipid antibodies and platelets or the linings of blood vessels. The end result is clots in the arteries (emboli, thrombi) and veins. Many cases of what was thought to be central nervous system lupus-induced strokes turned out to be due to APL related clots. In the veins, APL patients have an increased incidence of phlebitis and pulmonary emboli. Several patients have only found out about APL when they repeatedly miscarried pregnancies. APL is not necessarily always associated with active SLE, and can be present independent of SLE. Even though steroid administration can lower APL blood levels, there is no evidence that this decreases coagulopathy risks.

How should APL be approached? First, every new lupus patient should have a VDRL (syphilis test), kaolin PTT (a clotting time specially primed to look for the anticoagulant), and anticardiolipin antibody performed. If necessary, other tests (Russell's viper venom test, other phospholipid antibody determinations) can be undertaken. We sometimes find that one test can be positive and the others negative. We recommend that all our patients with positive antibodies at potential risk take one baby aspirin a day as prophylaxis. This form of therapy has not been studied in a controlled fashion, but most rheumatologists have had few adverse outcomes with this form of treatment. Any patient who develops thromboemboli while on low dose aspirin should be considered to be a candidate for long-term anticoagulation with coumadin (if venous) or subcutaneous heparin (if arterial). Patients with low platelet counts often need corticosteroids, but steroids do not help acute thromboembolic episodes unless they are also associated with active disease. Central nervous system manifestations of APL are treated with anticoagulation and platelet antagonists as opposed to steroids. Women who are recurrent aborters can be managed with baby aspirin, and if necessary, subcutaneous heparin while pregnant.

The next few years will see many new breakthroughs in this area. The Lupus Foundation of America is funding APL research programs that should help us better understand this recently described entity.

Blacks and Lupus

By Stanley Ballou, M.D.

It has been known since the early 1900's that systemic lupus erythematosus (SLE, lupus) is much more common in women than in men and that most women who develop this disease are in the middle adult years, usually between 20 and 40. It was not realized until the pioneering epidemiologic studies of Siegel and colleagues in 1955, however, that lupus is more common in black persons than in caucasians. Their studies, carried out in New York City and Jefferson County, Alabama, suggested that lupus was about three times as common in blacks as in whites. Most other studies of the occurrence of lupus have confirmed these findings. In a large study in San Francisco, Fessel observed that lupus was present three times as commonly in black people as in whites. Data from Cleveland and Baltimore also confirm that lupus is perhaps two to three times more common in blacks than whites. Unfortunately, there is not enough data available to determine whether lupus is a more common illness in blacks from other countries, particularly Africa.

It is of interest that similar studies of the occurrence of lupus have found that the disease also seems to be more common in several other races, including orientals and possibly hispanics, than in caucasians.

The reason why lupus appears to be more common in american blacks is not known. Although one might wonder whether lupus is more common in black people for socioeconomic reasons, the studies carried out in New York City found no evidence that socioeconomic factors were related to the occurrence of lupus. Nor have there been data from any other parts of the country to suggest that the cause of lupus is linked to any particular social or economic class of individuals.

Recently, it has been found that certain inherited genes are present more commonly than expected in persons with lupus. This finding indicates that heredity may play a role in the cause of lupus, and suggests that the increased occurrence of lupus in blacks (and perhaps other races) may be related to heredity. It is hoped that the research currently being carried out in this country, as well as in people of different races in other countries, will help to determine whether particular inherited genes account for the different frequency of lupus in different races.

Although we don't know why lupus is more common in blacks, we know that this is an important problem, because loss of life due to lupus (mortality) appears to be higher in blacks than in whites. This is probably not because lupus is a more severe illness in blacks, but because it is just more common in black persons. Nevertheless, the substantial mortality of lupus in blacks indicates that this is a major public health issue. Because of this a number of steps have been taken to increase public awareness of lupus in blacks and to promote research in this area. Two government task forces have recently focused on lupus in the black population. In addition, studies are being carried out to determine the frequency of persons with undiagnosed and untreated lupus in the black community. Finally, a number of community and public service efforts are underway to increase awareness of lupus nationwide. All of these efforts should serve to focus public and professional attention on the occurrence of this potentially serious disorder in American blacks, and in other minority races in America and perhaps in various races throughout the world. We hope that this increased awareness will lead to improved diagnosis and perhaps to earlier and more effective treatment for all persons with lupus erythematosus.

The Impact of Race in SLE

By John D. Reveille, M.D.

As the various abnormalities of the immune system that are seen in systemic lupus erythematosus (SLE) become more clear and newer treatments are identified, increasing interest is being focused on the role of factors such as heredity and race on the course and prognosis of this disease. It has been known for nearly 15 years that SLE was most common in american black women. Some studies have shown the blacks have a worse prognosis, thought to be due to more serious lupus manifestations such as kidney involvement or to socioeconomic factors. Other reports have disputed this, although they were usually examining small numbers of patients.

In order to critically determine the role of race in the presentation of SLE, we recently looked at differences in clinical features and prognosis in SLE in approximately equal numbers of american black and caucasian patients. (203 and 184, respectively). We found that black SLE patients tended to be much younger than caucasians when they developed lupus. Furthermore, the female predominance that is well described in this disease was much greater in black than in causasians. The tendency to develop skin rashes on exposure to sunlight, a well described phenomenon we know as photosensitivity, was much more common in caucasians, although the scarring rashes of lupus, known as discoid lupus, were slightly more frequent in american black patients. Kidney disease in SLE is an especially feared complication, often requiring large doses of prednisone or prednisone-like medications, or even stronger medicines. We found that kidney involvement in american black patients was considerably more common than in caucasians. We also discovered, as have other investigators, that those with lupus beginning at an early age, such as in the teens or early twenties, were much more likely to have their kidneys affected by SLE. Since american blacks tended to be much younger at onset of lupus, this at least in part explained the greater likelihood for american black patients to develop kidney disease.

When the prognosis in SLE was determined in our study, blacks tended to do worse than caucasians. The reasons for this are not completely clear. Some have blamed this on socioeconomic factors. However, this did not seem to be a significant factor in our study. Clearly the increased frequency of kidney disease could be one reason. But even when we corrected for this, blacks did worse than caucasians. Others have blamed the worse prognosis in american blacks on lesser access to medical care. However, the time elapsed between the onset of symptoms and diagnosis of SLE by a physician was actually less in blacks than in caucasians. Thus, other factors seem to be at work. However, what these additional things were that worsened the prognosis in blacks is not entirely clear. Whether such other complicating factors as hormones, or educational status or other things in the environment are contributing to this can only be speculated, and should be studied further.

There is a lot that we can thus do with this information. Since SLE is more common in blacks, and since the prognosis seems to be worse in this racial group, attempts at better education about lupus and its treatment should be especially aimed at young blacks, the group with the highest frequency of SLE and worse complications thereof. Other factors involved in predispositions to lupus such as heredity or environmental triggers should especially be studied in this group. SLE is a disease that transcends all racial and ethnic groups, and by helping to improve the course and prognosis in the higher risk groups we will ultimately be working for the betterment of all patients with SLE.

SLE in Males versus Females: Is There A Difference?

By M.B. Urowitz, M.D., FRCP

Systemic lupus erythematosus is an uncommon disorder in men, the sex ratio being in the order of 9 females to one male. Information suggesting that sex hormones modify susceptibility to the expression of SLE and some reports of the concurrence of SLE and Klinefelter's Syndrome, (XXY), raised two questions: (1) Is SLE in males the same as in females? and (2) Are affected males different from unaffected males with respect to their "maleness" and sex hormone profile? These questions were addressed in a study of 51 male patients followed at the Wellesley Hospital SLE Clinic in Toronto. In order to compare the clinical aspects of male and female SLE, 50 age and disease duration-matched female controls were selected for comparison.

Results of Investigations

1. Clinical Comparison of SLE in males and females.

The two populations of patients studied had a similar mean age, of diagnosis of lupus, and duration of follow-up. There was the same incidence of caucasians, blacks and orientals. A large number of clinical and laboratory characteristics of SLE were examined in both groups of patients and there was no obvious difference between the two groups in this analysis. Therefore the clinical presentation of SLE in males was similar to females.

2. Disease Severity Assessment.

The question as to whether the disease was more severe in men or women was examined in a number of ways. The mean number of ARA criteria as possible manifestations were enumerated in both groups, and the mean number of the severe manifestations, such as renal, neurologic, or vascular involvement were enumerated separately. As well, the number of patients with permanent renal or neurologic damage were tabulated. Complications such as osteonecrosis and major infections were examined in both groups as well as the amount of medication used. In all of these comparisons there was no difference between males and females, and therefore disease severity was similar in both groups of patients.

Clinical and Laboratory Assessment of "Maleness"

Fifty of the 51 male patients all had normal male characteristics without any evidence of feminization at all. The one patient with Klinefelter's syndrome (XXY) had the characteristics of that condition. Thirty-two of the men had offspring and for most of the others the lack of offspring had easy explanation. Buccal smears looking for chromosomal evidence of "maleness" were normal male in all of the male patients studied. In hormone studies the men generally had depressed plasma testosterone levels, and this finding was also reported by the Mexican unit in April of 1987. This finding might be related to the use of corticosteroids for the treatment of lupus and likely does not result in a loss of testosterone activity. On the other hand, a significant proportion of the men had elevated plasma estrogen levels, which was again confirmed by the Mexican group in 1987. This of course raises the possibility that increased estrogen levels in these patients may facilitate the development of lupus, as it has done in the mouse model of this disease.

In summary then, one can conclude that typical SLE with all of the usual clinical associations occurs in clinically and chromosomally normal men. Secondly, many of these men have elevated plasma estrogen levels which may have some pathogenic and therapeutic importance.

Sun Exposure and the Lupus Patient

By Stephen E. Ullrich, Ph.D.

The sun is essential for all life on this planet. Primitive cultures were aware of this and primitive peoples often worshipped the sun. Even during the Middle Ages, the momentary "absence" of the sun during a solar eclipse was a terrifying event. Why is it then, that on the eve of the 21st century, we advise lupus patients to avoid the sun? Because lupus is an autoimmune disease and the harmful ultraviolet (UV) radiation found in sunlight can adversely affect the regulation of the immune system.

The primary function of the immune system is to protect the host against microbial infections. One of the major weapons in the immune arsenal responsible for killing infectious agents is the antibody molecule. Normally, antibodies are like guided missiles that bind to and destroy bacteria in a highly selective and specific manner. In an autoimmune disease such as lupus, autoantibodies are formed. The guidance system of autoantibodies is faulty. Rather than seeking out and destroying foreign invaders such as bacteria, autoantibodies seek out and destroy "self", the cells and tissues of your own body. One of the major characteristics of lupus is the formation of a variety of autoantibodies, particularly anti-nuclear antibodies. The targets of the anti-nuclear autoantibodies are usually found deep within the cells, in the nucleus, where they are inaccessible to attack. One reason that lupus patients are advised to stay out of sunlight is because UV radiation appears to alter the location of the targets of the anti-nuclear autoantibodies in skin cells. Exposing skin cells to low to moderate doses of UV radiation causes movement of the targets from deep within the cell to the surface, where they become accessible to attack by the anti-nuclear autoantibodies. The autoantibodies bind to the targets now on the surface of the skin cells and kill the cells. This may explain why sunlight accentuates the skin lesions and facial rash seen in lupus patients.

In higher doses UV is toxic, by itself it will kill cells. A sunburn is visual evidence of cellular damage caused by UV radiation. As a result, the cells break apart and the contents of the cells, including the nuclear targets of the autoantibodies, such as DNA, are released. The anti-nuclear autoantibodies bind to the DNA and form DNA-antibody complexes. These complexes are carried through the blood and deposited in the kidneys and joints and are instrumental in the development of the kidney damage and arthritis seen in some lupus patients. By damaging cells and causing the release of the target DNA into the blood stream, UV promotes the formation of antibody-DNA complexes.

UV radiation is also a carcinogen and is the primary cause of skin cancer. While it is prudent for everyone to minimize their exposure to UV radiation, it is especially important for lupus patients to avoid the UV radiation found in sunlight. In addition to being a carcinogen, UV radiation also suppresses the immune response, and studies using mice have demonstrated a close association between the immunosuppressive effects of UV radiation and its ability to produce skin cancer.

Because UV radiation is immunosuppressive, at first glance you may think that anything that suppresses the immune response would be beneficial in treating an autoimmune disease such as lupus. This, however, is not true with UV radiation because of the types of immune reactions suppressed by UV. Unlike the immunosuppressive drugs used to treat lupus, UV exposure does not inhibit the production of the autoantibodies, but rather suppresses other types of immune reactions such as anticancer immunity and some types of antibacterial immune reactions, thus predisposing patients to skin cancer development and perhaps increasing the chance for bacterial and viral infections.

Fortunately small changes in your lifestyle can help minimize your exposure to UV radiation. Avoid the most intense sunlight during mid-day (noon to 3:00 p.m.). Wear protective clothing, especially broad-brimmed hats to protect your face. Use a sunscreen with a minimum SPF (sun protection factor) of 15 to protect your skin from the harmful effects of UV radiation. Remember that early detection and treatment is the key to fighting cancer, and skin cancer is the easiest type of cancer to detect. Get into the habit of self examination. Look for changes, reddish patches or irritated areas of skin that don't heal, bleed or have uneven, raised or crusty borders. Pay close attention to moles. If they change color, increase in size or if their borders become uneven and scalloped, see your dermatologist. Also remember that although lupus makes you more susceptible to the harmful effects of UV radiation, everyone should restrict their sun exposure. Make sure that your kids and other family members are putting on hats and sunscreen. Get everyone involved in detecting the early signs of skin cancer. And leave the mid-day sun to mad dogs and Englishmen.

A Medical Visit to China
After Tiananmen Square

By Robert G. Lahita, M.D., Ph.D.

As part of a medical academic exchange I was invited to visit mainland China shortly after the Tiananmen Square events. This gave the Chinese an opportunity to learn a little bit more about my experience in the West with the disease lupus. Our plan was to visit hospitals and medical schools, and to lecture and round with Chinese physicians. The trip was almost derailed by the Tiananmen Square debacle. Nevertheless, we agreed to go after vigorous correspondence with physicians and we were assured that the current climate for academic exchange was as good now as in the past. Many of my colleagues in rheumatology and immunology have asked about Chinese medicine and its 6,000 year history and I have been fascinated by Chinese medicine for several decades. Some of these questions were whether the disease systemic lupus erythematosus was as common in mainland China as believed, whether rheumatoid arthritis was as prevalent as lupus or RA in the Western countries, and the extent to which AIDS and lyme arthritis were Chinese problems. I wondered just how the Chinese — known for their expediency — handled the diagnosis, treatment, and long-term care of lupus patients and how their treatment varied from that found in the West. Included in this fascination was the use of traditional medicine in the treatment of these disorders. In essence this was a trip to mysterious China to pursue the Eastern approach to diseases that confound the best clinicians in the West. This was too much of an adventure to bypass even in troubled times.

The Chinese in Singapore

China was well represented at the Singapore Conference on Lupus despite the political unrest of the previous spring and summer. We were able to glimpse for the first time new clinical data, which was presented in a fashion both technically adequate and simple. Studies of 35,000 employees of a factory who were tested for the appearance of autoantibodies like ANA were present. These were hardly data that could be amassed over a long time by even the most prodigious worker in any Western country. Confidentiality, institutional review board regulations, animal rights, and intellectual modesty seemed to have no place in a country where diligence, data and expediency were synonymous with pure "progress". The Chinese are endearing people and apologies for humble graphics always preceded a talk. The speakers were polite and modestly fluent in English. Problems only came after the talk with the usual technical questions associated with any provocative presentation. At these times our Chinese colleagues had to search for the appropriate words and phrases to defend data or clarify points of interest. No one scientist could fathom or understand the meaning of such data in the context of Singapore. In retrospect a trip was required to fully understand medicine in the context of China. A third world experience is a "must" for every clinician who wants a perspective on progress. This is particularly true of lupus.

Lecturing — an exercise in endurance

On our arrival in Guangzhou we were given some 30 minutes to unwind before we were hustled off to the host hospital to give the first talk. The host was Dr. De Qing Xu, a noted dermatologist and SLE expert. On my arrival on a Sunday afternoon, I found a very respectful and quiet crowd of about 200 people. There were the usual polite handshakes and greetings from all of those to whom I was introduced. I asked, "How long do I have?" Two hours only and about 30 minutes for questions. After my lengthy talk, made more so by the frequent pauses for the interpreter, questions were asked. No one left the hall until I finished answering the last one. Many of those in the audience who were not fluent in English asked excellent prepared questions which they read from notes.

Throughout the visit I spoke with an interpreter; the only exception was one group at the Peking Union Medical College in Beijing. In that talk, which I suspect was really an English exercise for the audience, I spoke on the effects of gender on the immune system and lupus, and the questions they asked at the end indicated that they had a fine command of English.

Hospitals — a new experience

The hospitals in China are something to see. We were given the "cook's tour" of some of the dingiest and most depressing institutions that I have ever seen. Sadly, the hospitals reminded me of our big urban hospitals back home. Our hosts continually reminded us about the poverty of China and the vast health care system which was available to all at little cost. Care in China hardly costs anything (a few dollars per day). It is probably the only health care system on earth where socialized medicine really works. Workers again get the best of what there is, but rooms were poorly lighted and often minimally heated. Water was usually everywhere because of the omnipresent heating boiler in the open hallway, which belched steam, leaked, should have been replaced years ago, and gave off little or no heat. Believe it or not, these sights were reminiscent of many floors in large New York City hospitals so they proved less shocking to us than they might have been for a visitor from a non-urban community hospital. The smell of the Chinese hospital was that of carbolic acid or phenol. This is a smell that I remember from the hospitals of my youth, this, the original antiseptic of Lord Lister. The ICU and the operating theaters though somewhat old — ancient by most standards — serve a busy mass of people who have little money and no expectation of comfort. They are in the hospital to get well and they were there for the long haul. One can understand why there are no DRG's or length of stay problems in China.

Some of the hospitals had special areas reserved for foreigners who might become ill during their travels. This surprised me since separation of all kinds of services for "foreigners" seemed to prevail throughout China.

Medical Practice — traditional and not

The practice of medicine in China is fine but paradoxical. There are Western medicine and traditional Chinese medicine under the same roof. In larger institutions there are large libraries that are well staffed, and the physicians read a great deal. There seemed to be few Western journals and since over 1,000 Chinese medical journals exist unavailable to the rest of the world, there is plenty to read. These journals, which boast circulations of from 500 to 100,000 are current in every specialty and are the mainstay of the Chinese medical library. I found at least two Chinese books about SLE and several Western tomes, including my own.

On the whole, medicines are not lacking in China — there is just less of a variety. Only one or two diuretics to give for edema. Nevertheless, some drugs, usually the generic varieties, are being made available by Western pharmaceutical corporations. They seemed quite knowledgeable about all sorts of agents with which I had no knowledge, and a few traditional agents were mixed in with the orthodox pharmacopoeia. A note about lupus therapy is in order here. The Chinese do use a great deal of prednisone, antimalarials, and cytoxan to treat SLE. Cytoxan seems less toxic in China, particularly to children, and consequently is used more frequently.

Traditional medicine in China is something that we have all heard about. To see it in practice is to experience something entirely different. Entire clinics and treatment areas are devoted to "acupuncture, moxibustion, and cupping" for everything from bronchitis to stroke. When conventional medicines fail and in some cases even when they don't, physicians call upon the traditionalists. Several universities exist in the large cities, which deal only with such forms of practice. These institutions train traditional physicians. The practice goes back thousands of years in some instances, and the Chinese delight in regaling foreigners with the merits of this or that procedure or potion. Acupuncture is well known in the West, but few of us have seen it practiced on large numbers of people. The dedicated staff of young physicians and nurse practitioners who place needles in hundreds of outpatients crammed into outpatient wards are a sight to see. Moxibustion or the burning of herbal medicines at the ends of strategically placed acupuncture needles offers a bizarre and equally unusual alternative to the "traditional" acupuncture. Cupping, an ancient art, was in full use in Beijing for the conditions from the common cold to bronchitis. The "science", which surrounds traditional medicine pervades Chinese practice. There are many worthwhile physical exercises in China that would probably do more for Western patients than some of the questionable unproven remedies conjured up by some of our contemporaries. The well-known Tai Chi exercises — widely practiced everywhere in China and in the West — is dwarfed by the mental and physical benefits of Chigong, an exercise based on the principles of acupuncture. Chigong is also purported to be a method of "strengthening" the immune system and of particular use in lupus patients. I could imagine this as the dawn of psychoimmunology in China!

Most interesting of all of these traditional therapies were the herbal medicines themselves. No one could adequately tell me exactly what was in 50cc syringes whose contents were artfully injected into hips, lumbar muscles, knees, chests, and virtually every part of the fleshy anatomy which lends itself to the storage and gradual distribution of all matter of substance. One agent which I was particularly fascinated with was an extract of *Tripterygium wilfordii* (a root from South China), which is said to have remarkable curative powers for rheumatoid arthritis, and other conditions like lupus renal disease. The exact nature of the herbal extract was not clear, not purified, and not available I was told because of demand. Nevertheless, I did learn that it was polyglycoside, which would someday be purified. I brought some home with me. I would suggest that a large Western pharmaceutical company invest in airfare to explore the nature of this compound which would undoubtedly be added to the list of effective immunosuppressants in the West.

The Chinese are inveterate epidemiologists. This observation is probably due to the fact that there are so many people to study and that they lend themselves for study. One might expect that a captive populous, which has to lend itself to numerous surveys and countless numbers of clinical assessments would protest, but the Chinese take such assessment in stride. I found that rheumatoid arthritis though common in China affects less than one percent of the population and that the female to male ratio is roughly 8 to 1. This in contrast to that seen in the West where the prevalence of the disease is 3-5% with a female to male ratio of 3 to 1. Lupus in China is much more common than in the West with a prevalence of 40-70 per 100,000 whereas in the West the prevalence is 10-40 per 100,000. We were repeatedly told that AIDS was non-existent in China with only five known cases, or at least five reported cases. Four of those were from travelers, I was assured, and one was from a transfusion. If drug abuse is present in China — which I am sure it is — then HIV has not ravaged the populous as it has here. I saw no HIV infection nor heard any discussion of it in any of the large urban hospitals which I visited.

141

We did hear about 150 cases of AIDS in one province of China from a New York Times report when we returned. One surprise to me was the description of Lyme disease in northern China. At least 40 cases have been reported in the far northeast. Deer and ticks exist in China and the *Borellia burgdorferii* organisms have been serologically identified. Lyme also exists in South China but there are no deer and thus no tick reservoir. The mode of transmission is unknown and may, according to the Chinese, be the mosquito.

This visit to mainland China gave us an opportunity to see medicine in a personal way, practiced in a land whose traditions go back 6,000 years and whose populous is one-third of the world's people. Lupus is a major problem in China and will be the subject of much investigation as this huge country changes. More expertise and technology is needed to explain the high prevalence of SLE, and doubtless it will come as China changes.

Lupus in China

In an exchange of letters with
Ming Jiang, M.D. and Liping Zhu, Ph.D.

In China, lupus is a commonly diagnosed connective tissue disease. According to a preliminary epidemiological survey in 1983, it prevalence is about 75 per 100,000 people. This means that there are over 750,000 SLE patients in our population. The ratio of men to women patients is about 1 to 7. Among the women patients, most of them are in their childbearing years, with an average age of 32.

It is well known that every organ of the body can be impaired by lupus and that the kidney is one of the most vulnerable organs. Based on the analysis of the clinical manifestations and the renal biopsies we found that about 9% of SLE patients had nephrotic syndrome as their primary symptom. Sometimes it is difficult to make a definite diagnosis of SLE patients as it may take up to nine years for the syndrome to manifest clearly. However, our accumulated clinical data have shown that the occurrence of renal involvement increases with prolongation of SLE history. At the onset of the disease, about 24% of the SLE patients show nephritis but four years after the onset as many as 92% of SLE patients may suffer from kidney damage. Although a renal biopsy demonstrated abnormal changes, some of the SLE patients had normal renal function. The disease in this category of patient is called subclinical lupus nephritis by us. However, its frequency is quite low. Among the 33 patients we have surveyed and diagnosed as lupus nephritis patients, only 2 belong in this category. No coronary arteriosclerosis was found in 8 of 9 patients we studied. In this regard, what we have found in China is quite different from what has been reported in Western countries. We have discovered 4 fatal cases of Libman-Sacks endocarditis involving the mitral valve. We have quite often come across SLE patients with small amounts of pericardial fluid. Ultrasonic cardiographical techniques have made it much easier to diagnose pericarditis. Most of these patients do not have much fluid and pericardial temponade is very rare. About 19% of SLE patients suffer from nervous system involvement, more often from central nervous system involvement, more often from central nervous system involvement. Their clinical manifestation is often characterized by epilepsy, paralysis and organic psychological disease. As for lung involvement, interstitial lung disease is common, with changes in the small airways. Lymph node enlargement is found in 35% of the patients. We have found 4 SLE patients with histocytic necrotizing lymphadenopathy (HNL), the pathologic change which is the same as that in the report of Kikuchi, a Japanese scientist. This means that SLE patients may suffer from HNL. Hence, we hold that HNL might not be an independent disease. Since corticosteroids are widely used in the treatment of SLE patients, infection is one of the most important causes of death; 45% of deaths were due to infection. Intravenous methylprednisolone pulse treatment (IV-MP) has been introduced and is helpful for some patients. Based on the experiences of the treatment in 36 patients we found that IV-MP is favorable for those SLE patients.

A Meeting With
Fu-Lin Tang, M.D.

On a recent visit to the Scripps Clinic and Research Foundation in La Jolla, California, I had the pleasure of meeting Dr. Eng M. Tan, head, Autoimmune Disease Center, at the Scripps Clinic. Dr. Tan showed me a letter he had recently received from Dr. Ming Jiang, Department of Medicine, Capital Hospital, Beijing, China. Dr. Ming Jiang wrote:

"SLE is a rather common disease in China. Last year I took care of about 120 cases of SLE in the outpatient clinic and in the ward. I am analyzing these clinical materials, particularly paying attention to the nervous, cardiac, renal, hepatic, lymph nodes, and hematologic manifestations in SLE separately. The 'Nervous System Involvement in SLE' has been summarized and submitted in press. The 'Heart Manifestation in SLE' will be completed soon. It revealed that Chinese SLE patients complicated with pericarditis were much lower (in number) than those in Western countries. Lymphadenopathy in SLE sometimes presented a necrotizing lymphadenitis with granulocytic infiltration."

Dr. Tan introduced me to Dr. Fu-Lin Tang, who had recently arrived from the Capital Hospital, in Beijing, People's Republic of China. Dr. Fu-Lin Tang is serving a research assistantship in studies on lupus in the NIAID-supported Allergic Disease Center at the Scripps Clinic Autoimmune Disease Center directed by Dr. Tan.

Dr. Fu-Lin Tang was holding in his hand the Chinese translation of *The Sun Is My Enemy*. He spoke of the great need for more public awareness and education about lupus throughout his vast country. Our National Public Relations Committee will make sure that lay literature will find its way to the lupus patients in China.

Lupus in Hungary

In Conversation with Laszlo Czirjak, M.D., Ph.D.

Our department is highly involved in the clinical and immunological investigations of the different connective tissue diseases.

Our special consultations are frequented by 270 patients with SLE. Furthermore, we treat 90 cases with progressive systemic sclerosis, 90 cases with mixed connective tissue disease, 50 patients with dermatomyositis-polymyositis syndromes and about 200 cases with Sjögren's syndrome and 300 patients with complicated rheumatoid arthritis or related diseases.

We are also involved in the education of the medical students and hold postgraduate courses in clinical immunology.

The Hungarian health care system is basically different from the American. Considering the costs, our health care system is virtually free for all Hungarian citizens. This situation, in fact, does not mean an equal chance for the diagnostic possibilities and treatment. Our care system for the patients with connective tissue diseases is relatively centralized. The great majority of the patients visit one of the few special Hungarian centers for regular consultation. This does not cause a significant problem because Hungary itself is a small Central European country.

Our department has 100 beds for the treatment of the severe cases and for diagnostic purposes. The basic laboratory tests including the determinations of anti-DNA, -SS-A, -SS-B, -Sm, -Rnp, -centromer autoantibodies, and the investigation of certain complement components are available in our department.

The 5-year survival of the patients with SLE is 88.6% and the 10-year survival is 81.4% in our department. Considering the symptoms, 53% of the patients with SLE showed renal involvement and 16% exhibited central nervous system manifestations. Among our patients there are 54 patients with old onset SLE. The lupus-like syndromes with the deficiency of complement components and the subacute cutaneous lupus erythematosus were found to be relatively rare conditions among

Hungarian patients.

Our scientific work focuses on the function of the monocytes and polymorphonuclear cells in the disease. We are also interested in the investigation of the different autoantibodies, including the lupus anticoagulant in SLE.

Personally, my responsibility is the treatment of patients with progressive systemic sclerosis. Our patients with progressive systemic sclerosis show some differences as compared to the American cases. The proportion of the male cases is extremely low. The exposure to chemicals, mainly to organic solvents, was shown in about 25% of the patients. We recently have emphasized the importance of the provoking environmental factors in the onset of the disease (Czirjak and Szegedi, 1987, Ann. Intern. Med. 107, 118.) Considering our scientific work, we demonstrated the increased metabolic activity of the polymorphonuclear neutrophil cells, which could contribute to the severe vascular endothelial injury in this disease. We also investigated the presence of anti-nuclear antibodies in the disease.

I spent a one-year period in Boston, MA. I worked in the Tufts University's Department of Pathology. I was involved in basic immunological research in the laboratory of M.J. Stadecker.

It was a great experience for me to learn of the well-organized American lupus and scleroderma associations. In the past, any patients' associations were very rare in Hungary. However, with the current political climate such Hungarian organizations are being formed, including one for patients with connective tissue diseases. Because of the small size of Hungary and the language difficulties, first we have started to organize an association for all patients with connective tissue diseases. At the present time the continuing education of the patients about their disease(s) is rather occasional in our country, therefore we need a well-organized patients' organization for this purpose.

Research In Bulgaria

By Emilia Spassova, M.D.

Dear Editor,

Since 1972, working as a hematologist and rheumatologist, I have been carrying on clinical on research and observation on SLE patients and their closest relatives. I have organized a dispensary clinic for such cases. For several years now I have been doing cytochemical peripheral blood tests of those patients. I am also looking for activities of the antiphospholipid syndrome clinically, as well as by proving the presence of circulating lupus anticoagulant and anticardiolipid antibodies. I am studying the early manifestations of brain vasculitis clinically, in the laboratory and by computer tomography of the brain.

I do my best to keep regularly in touch with the available medical publications on those problems. I would appreciate very much, if it is not much trouble for you, if you could send me some further medical publications on the stated above problems and on SLE in general.

More News From Hungary

By Laszlo Czirjak, M.D., Ph.D.

I have some good news, Dr. Czirjak wrote. The association for the patients with connective tissue diseases has just been formed. As a first step we decided to form an association for patients with SLE, PAA and dermato-, polymyositis. The patients leadership will send you a letter in the near future.

As we discussed in Boston, we would be happy if you could find time to visit Hungary next year. Your experience will be tremendous to our new organization.

Thank you very much for the publication of our paper in the *Lupus News*.

Besides, our department has made an important decision. With regard to our scientific life, we would like to establish a much closer relationship with the Western World. Towards this end we have decided to organize a symposium next May in Debrecen on the pathophysiological, immunological and clinical aspects of systemic sclerosis. We feel we should prepare ourselves for the World Congress Immunologist in Hungary, 1992.

Pro. Szegedi, the head of our department, is the general secretary of the Hungarian Society for Immunology. He also sends you his best regards and hopes he will meet you personally in Debrecen.

Voice Of America

An Interview With Brian Cislak

Over the past 8 years, Brian Cislak, Medical Editor of the Voice of America, has interviewed medical investigators, clinicians and lupus patients to bring public awareness and education about systemic lupus erythematosus throughout the world. The mail that follows after each broadcast exceeds all expectations! Literally, hundreds of letters are pouring in from the most remote corners of the world. Many of these letters are written by lupus patients, who now feel less isolated and less alone. These broadcasts have also increased the LFA's CFC funding from abroad.

Here are some excerpts from the latest interview with Arthur M. Krieg, M.D., senior staff fellow at the National Institute of Arthritis and Musculoskeletal and Skin Disease, and Henrietta Aladjem, a Founder of the Lupus Foundation of America, Inc. and Editor of *Lupus News*.

Dr. Krieg stressed that the immune system was developed over the course of evolution as a way of the body to protect itself from infections. "It was all very wonderful" Dr. Krieg said, "except for the problem when the immune system gets confused, and attacks the body's own tissues, thinking that they are invading organisms. Lupus," he said, "is an autoimmune disease: instead of just fighting infections as it is supposed to, it attacks the body's own tissue. It can attack any tissue in the body, which is why we call it a systemic disease. Among the organs that can be damaged by lupus are the joints, the skin, which can result in rashes of various types and, in some cases, even the brain." He stressed that lupus affects principally women of childbearing age, although about 10 percent of its victims are men. "It is believed," he said, "that lupus is three times more prevalent in black women than in white women. Lupus patients have one very important thing in common — difficulty in getting their condition properly diagnosed."

This is what Dr. Krieg said about the research he is in research involved in at the NIAMS:

"Our current research includes trying to identify some of

the genes that cause lupus so that we might be better able to treat it. One class of genes that particularly interests us are called endogenous retroviruses. A retrovirus is a type of small virus; endogenous retroviruses are non-infectious retrovirus-like genes that are inherited. Endogenous retroviruses have been present in all humans for many thousands of generations. Humans and mice with lupus make autoantibodies that bind to retroviral proteins. This suggests to us that endogenous retroviruses could trigger autoimmunity by making proteins that the immune system would mistake for those of a foreign retrovirus, and thus attack. Since these endogenous retroviral proteins are expressed on many of the regulatory cells in the immune system, any attack on the protein could interfere with normal immune regulation, perhaps resulting in autoimmunity.

Henrietta Aladjem spoke about her personal involvement in lupus and her long-lasting remission, that has been extended over twenty years. She spoke at length about the lupus fatigue, which does not really relate to fatigue as physicians and the public understand it.

"It is fatigue," she said, "that absorbs the whole person. It absorbs your feelings and your thinking." She recalled being in her thirties and feeling as if she had reached the age of ninety. "There are times when one can get really depressed coping with this fatigue," she said, "especially since nobody can understand how difficult it can be some mornings, when one does not have the strength to reach for a glass of water to take an aspirin."

Mrs. Aladjem described the National Lupus Foundation as a national, patient-oriented health organization. She pointed out that the LFA fundraises for research, educational programs and patient care. She said that while doctors are trying to delve into complicated scientific projects to find some answers, the LFA is trying to improve the quality of life of the lupus patient.

Our comments were heard in forty countries around the world. The LFA is grateful to Brian Cislak – and to the Voice Of America – for helping us year after year in bringing a measure of hope, where there was no hope before.

8

LUPUS AND THE GOVERNMENT

An Interview with Louis W. Sullivan, M.D., Former Secretary of Health and Human Services*

During my brief meeting with Secretary Louis W. Sullivan, M.D., his expression was warm; and he had a wide, radiant smile that was reflected in his eyes. His demeanor seemed the expression of a natural kindness, but there was something else as well. I had the feeling of having encountered a man who understands the needs of those who seek his help, and I was sure that he intends to help them.

I asked Secretary Sullivan the following questions:

Question: How can our government help, not only to increase the funding for biomedical research and lupus but also to help us promote public awareness and education so that we can reach all the minority groups in this country and all the patients who are perhaps not diagnosed, misdiagnosed, or even being treated with the wrong medications. How can we get help to do a better job, Dr. Sullivan?

Answer: Lupus is a very serious disease that affects a significant number of Americans, primarily young women and, in particular, black women. Our data indicate that, in terms of lupus, black women have a threefold higher incidence (number of new cases), prevalence (total number of cases), and mortality than whites. Public awareness and education are vitally important in combating this disease.

The National Institutes of Health (NIH) and the Office of Minority Health are working to increase public awareness. The NIH's National Institute of Arthritis and Musculoskeletal and Skin Diseases (NIAMS) has convened a task force to recommend new strategies and design educational materials specifically for minority audiences. The Office of Minority Health serves on this body.

In recent years, there has been a striking decrease in mortality from lupus. Today 95 percent of people with lupus survive ten years after diagnosis, compared with a 60 percent survival rate in 1965. Since 1965, lupus has become better recognized; and new serologic tests are providing important markers that allow physicians to target management of the disease to the individual patient. The NIH has played an important role in this effort.

Question: There is also a great need to study blacks in Africa, the Caribbean, and other such places. The physicians would like to know what the incidence of lupus is in these places. What would be the way to get some information about that?

Answer: NIAMS staff are making efforts to encourage research on SLE in minority populations and are making efforts to encourage research in this area. In 1987, the NIAMS issued a nationally distributed program announcement entitled "Clinical and Epidemiologic Research on Minority Populations of the United States" to encourage additional research in this area. Lupus is one of the diseases specified in the announcement. The minority populations to be studied include, but are not limited to, Blacks, Hispanic Americans (Mexican Americans, Puerto Ricans, Cuban Americans), Asian Americans, native Americans, and Pacific Islanders. The Institute is considering reissuing this ongoing program announcement.

One approach for gathering population-based data on lupus is exemplified in a study conducted in Baltimore, Maryland. An estimate of the incidence for specific sex-race groups and the total population was ascertained, based on first hospital discharge diagnosis, for a period of eight years. A similar study might be feasible in some parts of Africa and the Caribbean where it would be possible to identify all treated or perhaps hospitalized lupus cases within a contained region.

A great deal of cooperation is needed by all health care providers within a contained geographic area to carry out this type of study. Also, ascertainment bias is a major concern of the United States study and certainly any study carried out in a developing country; that is, individuals with lupus who are not receiving medical care or not correctly diagnosed are not identified in this study design. Therefore, there could be a very significant amount of underreporting of cases.

Question: As I have already indicated, investigators have good reasons to suspect that lupus is more severe in blacks. It would be important to know how severe lupus is in other countries. The physicians believe that it might be a severe disease. How can we help in this direction to have more accurate statistics at hand?

Answer: Many factors must be addressed in studies of lupus in high risk populations. Racial differences in the severity, age at onset, and outcome of systemic lupus erythematosus are poorly understood. In addition to genetic differences, certain environmental factors have been suggested to be associated with the disease or its severity: diet, exposure to physical agents, use of drugs, access to health care, lifestyle, and social factors related to socioeconomic status.

Question: It is well known that lupus with hypertension is a bad combination of diseases. This is particularly important to blacks because hypertension is an important health problem among the black population. This points to the same need for more public awareness and education. Again, how can we convey to our government the great need for help in this direction?

Answer: Through NIH and the Office of Minority Health, we are developing information specifically targeted to black women at risk for lupus. In addition, through the NIH's National Heart, Lung, and Blood Institute, there is a major national coordinated effort — the National High Blood Pressure Education program — to inform and educate the public concerning hypertension. This program includes activities directed at black populations.

Question: Dr. Peter H. Schur (Professor at Harvard Medical School and Director of Lupus Research at Brigham and Women's Hospital, in Boston) feels that there is a great need to determine accurately the prevalence of lupus (discoid lupus, systemic lupus erythematosus, and drug induced lupus). Furthermore, more accurate information is needed in reporting both the frequency and severity of these three lupus diseases in different ethnic populations and in caucasians. Making lupus a reportable disease would facilitate this investigation. The LFA supports these steps. Again, Dr. Sullivan, how can we make our government respond to our needs?

Answer: I agree that there is a need for more accurate statistics on the prevalence of lupus in various populations. In addition to the efforts mentioned in response to question 2, NIAMS staff have been working with the staff of the National Center for Health Statistics (NCHS) to incorporate lupus questions in their national surveys. The National Health and Nutrition Survey III, which is now being carried out by NCHS, does include the question: "Has a doctor ever told you that you have lupus?" Since the survey will have a higher proportion of blacks in the sample than in the United States population as a whole, it is hoped that some usable data will result.

Question: Several years ago, SSA started to draft new listings of diseases for purposes of determining eligibility of Social Security Disability benefits. These new listings, including a listing for systemic lupus erythematosus, were never released. What can you do to assist in the updating of the listings, which will help disabled individuals to obtain disability benefits? What are your comments, Dr. Sullivan?

Answer: It is true that SSA met with a panel of experts and that the panel made recommendations for revisions to the present listing for systemic lupus erythematosus to make it more specific. It should be noted, however, that while the current listing is rather brief, it effectively identifies those individuals who can be assumed to be disabled because of lupus. While the present listing is adequate to properly determine disability for individuals with lupus, Social Security is in the process of publishing a regulation based upon the panel's recommendations.

Question: The Medicare Catastrophic Coverage Act expanded Medicare benefits to include coverage for more hospital and skilled nursing care as well as including expanded drug and outpatient coverage for home health care. Shouldn't ill and disabled individuals be able to receive a broad range of nursing and other home health services without having to go to a nursing home? What can you do to expand the scope of Medicare home health coverage?

Answer: The Department is responsible for administering the Medicare home health care benefit within the limits defined by Congress. On the one hand, the benefit has expanded greatly in recent years, with the amount of Medicare outlays tripling during the past decade. On the other hand, the most recent revisions of the benefit enacted as part of the Medicare Catastrophic Coverage Act do not address what is often perceived as an inherent inequity: that those who need the most care, i.e., extended daily home care, do not qualify for it under terms of the current benefit. The catastrophic law does contain a provision establishing an advisory committee mandated to study various aspects of the current home health care provision and to report its findings to Congress.

Editor's note: Medicare benefits under the Catastrophic Coverage Act were repealed by Congress in November 1989.

Question: The spiralling cost of health care is one of our country's biggest problems. Many chronically ill individuals cannot afford to pay for their health care and cannot purchase insurance. What are you doing to control health care cost increases? What can health care consumers do to help in this process? Furthermore, many lupus patients are denied health insurance because their lupus is a pre-existing condition. Lupus is a very costly disease to treat; and as mostly young women have this disease, it means years of treatment and medication for these patients. How are they supposed to pay for it?

Answer: There is a widespread recognition today that, even though the best medical care in the world is available in the United States, our health care system is not serving all our citizens in the way it should. America's health care financing system needs a top-to-bottom review if it is to continue to live up to the expectations of our citizens. If we are going to keep the best in American health care, improve access to care, and, at the same time, keep health costs in line, we are going to have to examine that most fundamental aspects of our health care system and look at many possibilities for change.

That process is already underway. The Congress created a special commission to look at chronic care needs, the Pepper Commission, and it will be making recommendations next March. In addition, I appointed the independent quadrennial Advisory Council on Social Security last June and asked that they look especially at our health care system, in particular the Medicare and Medicaid programs, which were created under the Social Security law.

Within HHS, I have also launched a comprehensive review of our national health and long-term care financing policies, which is being directed by HHS Under Secretary Constance Horner. I have specifically asked that this review look at fundamental, long-term reforms of public and private health care financing that may be necessary to improve access for the poor, minorities, and the uninsured, or other population groups which are disadvantaged by current policies and programs. The review will also look at Medicaid in particular.

In addition, I want to find better ways to bring about a public and private sector partnership, as well as increasing the participation of the private sector in financing long-term care.

I think that the main point is that people now recognize that our health care system needs more than band-aids or even minor health surgery to address the joint problems of quality, access, and costs. We are not looking for quick or easy fixes. We are looking at the fundamentals of our existing systems to find what changes are needed to maintain a health care system of the highest quality which serves all our citizens fairly without breaking the bank.

Question: As it now stands, the Social Security Administration does not recognize chronic fatigue as a symptom for disability. Most lupus patients suffer from an incredible fatigue and exhaustion and frequently are denied payments from SSA. (The Veterans Administration changed its description of lupus last summer and now recognizes lupus patients as suffering from fatigue.) Can SSA change its requirements concerning fatigue? This is truly important.

Answer: Fatigue is considered in making a determination of disability for persons with lupus in the same manner as it is considered for other impairments. The symptom of fatigue, along with the signs and laboratory findings, is evaluated to determine that degree of severity of the impairment.

In some situations, an individual's symptoms, such as fatigue, suggest the possibility of a greater restriction of the individual's ability to function than can be demonstrated by the objective medical evidence alone. In such cases, other information, such as the individual's activities of daily living, the extent of activity before fatigue occurs, the frequency at which the individual requires periods of rest, etc., is considered in conjunction with the medical evidence. From all this information, a reasonable conclusion is drawn regarding the individual's ability to work.

Question: The House has already passed an appropriation asking for a $3 million increase in funding for NIAMS, specifically mentioning lupus. Dr. Sullivan, will you help us in convincing the Senate Subcommittee on Health to do likewise?

Answer: The President's fiscal year 1990 budget request for the National Institute of Arthritis and Musculoskeletal and Skin Disease is $169 million. Within that budget, research on lupus is an important priority. In 1988, NIAMS spent nearly $11 million for research on lupus, and that effort will continue as new project applications are reviewed and approved.

I'll attempt to see the Secretary again and perhaps have more time with him so that I can explain in greater detail to him the plight of the lupus patient.

Note: The Editor would like to acknowledge the assistance of Deborah Thomson, J.D., in the preparation of questions for this interview. *HHS News.*

HHS NEWS
U.S. Department of Health and Human Services

Statement by Louis W. Sullivan, M.D.

The Lupus Foundation of America's initiative to educate minority Americans about systemic lupus erythematosus and its warning signs is a most important endeavor. To that end, my Department is working with the Foundation to develop materials to reach these groups, including translation of education literature into Spanish. Our efforts at HHS will complement the work of the Lupus Foundation in carrying out its nationwide minority outreach campaign.

*I was helped with some of the questions for this article by Deborah Thompson, J.D.

159

An Interview with Otis Bowen, M.D., Former Secretary of Health and Human Services*

O tis R. Bowen, M.D., is a family physician who has practiced medicine most of his life in the small town of Bre-
men, Indiana. He has combined his career as a doctor
with that of public servant, and he is the first physician to
serve as Secretary of Health and Human Services. His term as
secretary has been marked, so far, by efforts to improve coverage for severe illnesses which result in catastrophically high
medical expenses.

I asked Dr. Bowen the following questions:

Question: What is the status of the Social Security disability
program's revision of the medical listing for SLE? When will
the new listing be released?

Answer: The Social Security Administration convened a
panel consisting of appropriate outside medical experts, rep-
resentatives of the state disability determination services that
make decisions on disability claims, and SSA medical and policy staff. This panel reviewed SSA's evaluation criteria for musculoskeletal impairments and connective tissue disease and
completed its review in December 1986. One of the panel's recommendations is to revise the listing for systemic lupus erythematosus. The recommended revision takes into consideration comments made by the Lupus Foundation of America
when the last revision of these listings was published in the
Federal Register on December 6, 1985.

SSA will now begin a study to determine the reliability and
administrative impact of disability decisions under the panel's
proposed revised listings. Publication of a Notice of Proposed
Rulemaking (NPRM) is scheduled for the spring of 1988. We
certainly invite LFA to comment on the proposed changes.
After public comments received on the NPRM are resolved,
SSA will publish a final rule.

Question: What provision does HHS plan to make for providing health insurance for patients in long-term care?

Answer: Through the Medicaid program, HHS and states already pay for a substantial portion of the long-term care provided to Americans — on the order of half the nation's total long-term care bill. However, Medicaid only becomes available as a payor of last resort when the patient's resources have been exhausted. Medicare also pays for some shorter-stay nursing home care, but the Medicare program was designed to cover acute care coverage, not long-term custodial care.

Many Americans are unaware that Medicare is not intended to cover long-term care, and one step that HHS must take is to better inform our beneficiaries so that they will not be caught by surprise if they should need this kind of care. At the same time, we are also encouraging private insurance companies to offer long-term policies. Until recently, private policies of this kind have been virtually unavailable. But today there is rapidly growing interest; and approximately 60 companies are in the long-term care insurance market, with more than 400,000 policies already purchased. I expect this market to continue to grow rapidly.

In addition, I have recommended that we make available a new IRA-type savings account, an "Individual Medical Account," in which people could save for possible long-term care expenses on a tax-advantaged basis. This proposal is under study by the Treasury Department.

Finally, of course, we do not want to sacrifice the home and community based care which has always been the most important kind of "long-term care." People want to stay in their homes and in the community, and we want to encourage that and do everything we can to make it possible.

Question: Do you favor national health insurance? If not, how do you propose to provide health care for uninsured persons?

Answer: Americans are well-served by a health insurance system that reflects the diversity of our needs. National health insurance would represent a centralized regulatory approach that would not serve us as well and would surely create new problems of its own.

Those who lack insurance, likewise, are not a single population but represent different groups with different problems. Therefore, we must seek a variety of solutions:

For the working poor, we must look to the employment relationship as a mechanism to secure greater access to insurance. This means a greater employer role and increased effort by the private insurance industry.

For the indigent, local and state governments have a historical and legal responsibility to provide for their health care needs. Local and state general medical assistance financing and free services programs, including public hospitals, are intended to meet those needs. In addition, such targeted Federal programs as Community Health Centers, the Health Services and Mental Health state grants, and hospitals' Hill-Burton obligations finance large amounts of care to indigent persons.

For families who are categorically eligible for Medicaid but have too much income, states already have the flexibility to change the basic income eligibility and spend-down thresholds so as to cover more people. Even without such a change, states have considerable latitude in electing which optional categories of people they wish to cover (for example, certain pregnant women).

For catastrophic insurance, several approaches — including the one the President has sent to Congress — are under discussion.

For persons with medical conditions for which they cannot obtain insurance at all or can obtain it only at a prohibitively high price, the states have demonstrated clear leadership in addressing this problem, especially through pooling of these risks. As of last year, six states had operational programs, four additional states' programs are expected to become operational in 1987, seventeen more states have considered legislation, and four states were conducting studies. States can tailor such programs to their particular circumstances, and I believe that this is the best approach. In addition, the Federal government is considering what types of support and technical assistance might be provided to states when they consider the development of such pools.

Question: Should employers be required by law to provide health insurance to their employees?

Answer: Health insurance for Americans is provided through a mixed and flexible system that allows for a great deal of accommodation to individual needs. While employment-based insurance is the dominant source of coverage, many have also secured insurance through such other means as individual enrollment in HMOs and private purchase of insurance tailored to their needs. This mixed system has worked well in making available the highest quality of care for

162

our citizens. While we certainly favor increased availability and holding of insurance products, including employment-based insurance, it is not clear that we would improve the system overall by mandating such coverage through Federal law in every employment situation. This would be a fundamentally new regulatory step; and the case for intrusion of this kind by the Federal government, with potentially severe effects on labor cost and employment, has not been made.

Question: Haven't Medicare DRGs resulted in lupus patients being discharged more quickly from the hospital, often in frail condition?

Answer: Under the prospective payment system, Medicare uses diagnosis related groups (DRGs) to pay hospitals a fixed cost per admission according to the patient's diagnosis, rather than the actual costs per admission. But the Medicare payment made to the hospital for a particular DRG does not determine the maximum time the patient may remain in the hospital. The only criteria for how long the patient remains in the hospital are whether further inpatient hospital care is medically necessary and whether the hospital is the proper place to provide care, regardless of the patient's diagnosis.

It is true that average length of stay has been declining; but this trend, which pre-dates PPS, has been under way for many years; and it results from changes in medical practice, not just DRGs. We do not have any evidence of a pattern of discharges that would be considered medically inappropriate. Medicare is committed to maintaining high quality care even while it encourages greater efficiency and cost effective care.

Question: Patients complain they can't get admitted into a hospital when they are sick with lupus because of DRG, etc., rules. Please comment.

Answer: When hospitalization is needed, Medicare is committed to making the proper care available. But as has always been the case with Medicare reimbursement for care, medical necessity and appropriateness of setting are not determined solely by diagnosis. Rather, the individual patient's condition as well as the services that he or she is going to receive or has received are taken into account in determining whether inpatient hospital services are medically necessary.

Decisions on hospital admission depend first on the patient's physician. In addition, Peer Review Organization reviewers, who must be actively practicing medicine in the PRO geographic area, may make determinations based on their own knowledge, experience, and training. They discuss the case with the attending physician before any denial determination is made. As this process suggests, PRO review is designed to consider existing medical conditions or circumstances of the Medicare patient when determining whether the admission is medically necessary and appropriate.

Question: Many lupus patients have optioned for HMOs because they are cheaper than Blue Cross/Blue Shield. Now many are complaining that the care they receive is second rate. What can be done to improve quality for all patients in HMOs?

Answer: Complaints regarding the quality of care provided by HMOs to their enrollees should initially be brought to the attention of the appropriate contact person identified by the individual HMO. In some instances, the quality problem may relate to a lack of understanding concerning the benefits provided by the HMO. And where there appears to be a problem with the services provided, the HMO is in the best position to investigate and determine how to make corrections and carry them out.

In addition, Congress recently enacted legislation providing for the ongoing review by Peer Review organization or other similar entities of the quality of care furnished by HMOs to their Medicare enrollees. The department issued a Request for Proposal on March 9, soliciting proposals in 25 states for the conduct of this review — in the remaining states the review will be assigned to the current PRO, the organization that is now reviewing the hospital care furnished to Medicare beneficiaries. The organizations conducting this review will be looking at medical records to determine whether there are quality problems at individual HMOs, and they will also serve as a point for any Medicare enrollee complaints regarding quality concerns.

Question: What can be done to educate the public regarding the futility and waste of money for quack cures, quack treatments, health food, extra (mega) vitamins, etc.?

Answer: We have had no inquiries regarding quackery involving lupus. However, along with the Postal Service and the Federal Trade Commission, my department, through the Food and Drug Administration, is on the alert for quackery. When the quackery threatens health, FDA moves through the Justice

Department to prosecute.

By and large, this readiness to act has successfully rid the United States of quack clinics with dangerous ineffective "cures" of the kind found in Mexico along the U.S. border, on some Caribbean islands, and in some European countries.

Through import alerts to Custom officials, FDA also bars quack products' being distributed in the United States from abroad.

FDA works closely with the Better Business Bureau nationwide as well as with heart, cancer, and arthritis groups, as well as others, to dispel myths and expose particular quackery scams through publications, background information, features, and news columns. FDA's press office is an aggressive clearinghouse of quackery information. Many of its columns and backgrounders suggest that people considering an unorthodox treatment check various sources, including volunteer health organizations, for their views.

Question: What can the PHS/NIH/NSF do to help find the cause/cure for lupus?

Answer: The NIH supports biomedical research on lupus through grants and contracts to universities and medical schools throughout the country, as well as conducting studies in laboratories on the NIH campus in Bethesda, Maryland.

Federally supported research on lupus is now quite extensive. In just the past few years, new data has emerged from research studies that have uncovered several diverse defects of the immune system; research on genetic and environmental factors that regulate the disease; studies of abnormal estrogen metabolism; evaluations of the course and the available treatments of the disease and its complications; and studies that are developing improved therapies, including drugs and other techniques.

A new publication on recent research is available: Update: *Lupus Erythematosus Research,* prepared by staff of the National Institute of Arthritis and Musculoskeletal and Skin Diseases, which discusses research progress toward conquering the disease.

Question: Till we find the cause and cure for lupus, what can we do to improve the treatment of lupus patients?

Answer: In order to improve the treatment of lupus patients, researchers are continuing to improve previous forms of treatment and to develop new ones. Additional new drugs that act to suppress the immune system and reduce the production of antibodies are being evaluated. Research has indicated that sex hormones may play an important role in the development of lupus. This suggests the possibility of sex hormone therapy.

In addition, investigators have shown that a diet rich in fish oil may be beneficial for lupus in experimental models of this disease. They showed that diet rich in eicosapentaenoc acid (EPA), a fatty acid in fish oil, protected female NZB/NZW mice, a mouse model of lupus, from developing lupus nephritis and greatly reduced mortality.

Future research on lupus will include the use of monoclonal antibodies that are directed against specific components of the immune system and the use of immune cell products, such as interferon or interleukin, that alter cell function.

*Deborah Thomson, J.D., helped me formulate some of my questions to Dr. Bowen.

Combined Federal Campaign Funds Result In Increased Foundation Services

By Jane Tado, Director of Federated Programs, L.F.A.

There is beginning to be substantial evidence among LFA Chapters that funds from the Combined Federal Campaign are making a considerable impact on program services, such as increased and diversified patient services and public education activities, and the ability to provide more funds for lupus research. Many chapters are now able to initiate services they have dreamed for years of providing.

Within the next few years, the Lupus Foundation of America hopes to move gradually into other federated campaigns, such as Combined Health Appeals and State and Municipal Employees Campaigns. Added revenue from these sources will mean more and better services for those with the disease, and an increased funding base for research to find the cause and cure for lupus.

GLOSSARY*

ANTIBODY: Serum protein made in response to an antigen.

ANTIGEN: Protein that stimulates formation of antibodies.

ANTINUCLEAR ANTIBODY TEST: Blood test to detect antibodies to nuclei.

ARTHRALGIA: Aches and pains in one or many joints.

ARTHRITIS: Inflammation in a joint with heat, swelling, pain, and redness.

ASPIRIN: In 1763, researchers discovered that an extract of the willow bark was effective in relieving the pains of rheumatism. Willow extract owes its therapeutic efficacy to a substance called salicylic acid — from the Latin name for willow, *salix*. A chemically modified form, acetylsalicylic acid, is marketed under the name of aspirin. For reasons still unknown, aspirin helps relieve pain and reduce inflammation.

AUTOANTIBODY: Antibody directed against the body's own tissue.

AUTOGENOUS VACCINES: Vaccines made from the patient's own bacteria, as opposed to vaccines made from standard bacterial cultures.

AUTOIMMUNE: Sensitive to one's self; a person's body makes antibodies against some of its own cells.

BASAL METABOLISM TEST: Determines whether the body's metabolism is over- or underactive.

BASOPHIL: One of the granulated white blood cells

BIOPSY: Sample of tissue taken for microscopic study.

BLOOD CELL: Three main kinds are recognized: red blood cells (erythrocytes) carry oxygen and carbon dioxide; white blood cells (leukocytes) help fight infection; platelets (thrombocytes) help prevent bleeding.

B LYMPHOCYTE (B CELL): Lymphocyte that makes antibodies.

BRONCHII: The tubes formed by the division of the windpipe, which convey air to the lung cells.

BUN: Blood urea nitrogen; when the kidneys fail, the BUN rises, as does the uric acid.

BUTTERFLY RASH: Form of double-wing-shaped skin rash around the nose and cheeks highly suggestive lupus.

CAPILLARIES: Smallest of the blood vessels that connect arteries and veins.

CELL BIOLOGIST: One who studies cell architecture and function.

CHRONIC: Lasting for a long period of time.

CNS: Central nervous system.

COLLAGEN DISEASE: Group of diseases characterized by inflammation of connective tissues, especially the skin and joints — rheumatoid arthritis, SLE, scleroderma, Sjögren's syndrome, juvenile rheumatoid arthritis — also usually synonymous with rheumatic disease.

COMPLEMENT PROTEIN: Regulatory molecule of the immune response.

CONNECTIVE TISSUE: Substance that binds the body together, like a body glue. Connective tissue is the most widespread and abundant tissue in the body.

CORTICOSTEROID: Product of adrenal cortex.

CORTISONE: Potent hormone of the adrenal glands; the pure compound was first discovered in adrenal secretion simultaneously in 1936 by Dr. Edward C.

Kendall of the Mayo Clinic, and by Dr. Reichstein of Basel, Switzerland. It is now synthesized as a pure chemical.

COVALENT: Chemical bond formed by the sharing of electrons.

CUTANEOUS LESIONS: Visible changes in skin that are abnormal; rashes, sores, or scars.

CYTOPLASM: Part of the cell that surrounds its nucleus.

DEOXYRIBONUCLEIC ACID (DNA): Basic constituent of genes. Genes are the cellular constituents that govern heredity. Deoxyribonucleic acid is a large, complex molecule composed of chemicals called sugars and nucleic acids.

DERMATOMYSOTIS: A chronic inflammatory disease of the skin and muscles.

DIPLOPIA: Double vision.

DISCOID LUPUS: Lupus confined to the skin and characterized by atrophy and scarring.

DIURETIC: A drug that helps to make more urine.

DROPSY: Swelling of the legs and abdomen that is most often caused by heart failure, but can be due to kidney or liver disease.

EKG (or ECG): Electrocardiogram, a recording of electrical forces from the heart.

ENDOCRINOLOGY: Study of the glands of internal secretion.

ENZYME: Protein substance that catalyzes a biological or chemical reaction.

ERYSIPELAS: Contagious, infectious disease of skin and subcutaneous tissue, marked by redness and swelling of affected areas and with constitutional symptoms.

ERYTHEMA NODOSUM: Painful red bumps on the skin; a skin manifestation of several diseases, but rarely of lupus.

ERYTHROCYTES: Normal nonnucleated red cells of the circulating blood; the red blood corpuscles.

ESTROGEN: Female hormone produced by the ovaries; it is responsible for secondary sexual characteristics in females and for the preparation of the uterus for implantation of the fertilized egg.

EXACERBATION: Recurrence of symptoms; another word for flare.

FALSE-POSITIVE SYPHILIS TEST: There are a number of tests for syphilis, including the Wasserman, RPR, Hinton, and VDRL tests. Some people will have a positive test for syphilis without having the disease. Systemic lupus erythematosus is one of the conditions that may give a positive test for syphilis, although syphilis is not present. This is called a false-positive test for syphilis. Lupus patients can make antibodies to a lipidlike (fatlike) substance structurally similar to the syphilis organism, and consequently may have a false-positive test for syphilis.

GALACTOSE: One of the sugars in milk, a part of the lactose molecule.

GASTRIC: Belonging to the stomach.

GASTRIC PARIETAL CELLS: Acid-producing cells of the stomach.

GENETIC: Pertaining to the genes; the word *genetic* refers to the property of transmission of parental characteristics to offspring. See DEOXYRIBONUCLEIC ACID.

GLOMERULONEPHRITIS: Type of kidney inflammation characterized by involvement of the glomerulus of the kidney.

HAPTEN: Chemical that will induce an immune response when coupled to a protein.

HEMATOLOGIST: Specialist in the study of blood.

HEMATURIA: Red blood cells in the urine.

HEMIPARESIS: Paralysis or weakness of one side of the body.

HEMOLYTIC ANEMIA: Condition characterized by a reduction in circulating red blood cells due to increased destruction of the cells by the body.

HEPATITIS: Inflammation of the liver.

HISTIOCYTE: Tissue macrophage — scavenger of cell debris, viruses, bacteria.

HISTOCOMPATIBILITY ANTIGEN (HLA): Cell-surface protein involved in transplant rejection; HLA proteins are controlled by genes on the sixth chromosome.

HISTOLOGY: Examination of tissue under a microscope as opposed to the gross clinical examination.

HISTOPATHOLOGY: Pathologic change in tissues and cells as seen under a microscope.

HLA SYSTEM: Genetic system controlling proteins on cell surfaces; often linked to disease.

HORMONE: From the Greek "to excite"; hormones are chemical messengers that excite a response in other tissue.

HYBRIDOMA: Fusion of an antibody-producing cell and a myeloma (tumor) cell that makes a great deal of monoclonal antibody.

HYDROXYCHLOROQUINE (PLAQUENIL): Antimalarial drug that has also been used as a treatment for lupus.

HYPERSENSITIVITY: Form of allergy generally mediated by antibodies.

HYPOCHONDRIAC: One who has morbid anxiety about health.

IMMUNE COMPLEXES: Specific combination of antibodies with their corresponding antigens.

IMMUNE RESPONSE: Response of the body's immune system to antigens.

IMMUNITY: Power to resist infection.

IMMUNOFLUORESCENCE: Special technique of histology using a fluorescent dye to mark antibody or immune process taking place at a given site in the tissue.

IMMUNOGEN: Any substance capable of eliciting immunity.

IMMUNOLOGIC TOLERANCE: Specific suppression of immunity to antigens. Normally, we do not make antibodies to our own antigens, such as our own cells, tissue proteins, or DNA.

LE CELL TEST: The LE cell is a white blood cell that has eaten the nucleus of another white blood cell; the latter appears as a blue-staining spot inside the first cell.

LYMPHOKINE: Proteins made by monocytes and lymphocytes that affect other lymphocytes.

LYSE: To produce disintegration of cells, causing them to release their contents.

MACROPHAGES: Tissue cells that eat antigens, complexes, bacteria, and viruses.

MAJOR HISTOCOMPATIBILITY MARKER: See HISTOCOMPATIBILITY ANTIGEN.

MEPACRINE (QUINACRINE, ATABRINE): Antimalarial drug that was taken by U.S. Armed Forces personnel during World War II.

METABOLISM: Series of chemical processes in the living body by which life is maintained.

METHYLPREDNISOLONE: Synthetic form of corticosteroid.

MIXED CONNECTIVE TISSUE DISEASE: Consisting of two or more of the connective tissue diseases, e.g., lupus, polymyositis, scleroderma.

MOTOR APHASIA: Loss of speech due to a brain defect affecting the muscles of speech.

MUCOSAL IMMUNITY: Immunity of the gastrointestinal, genitourinary, or bronchial tracts.

MYASTHENIA GRAVIS: Disease in which nerve impluses are not properly transmitted to the muscle cells; as a result, muscles all over the body become weak.

NAPROXEN (NAPROSYN): One of several nonsteroidal antiinflammatory drugs (NSAIDs).

NATURAL KILLER CELL: Cell that kills (lyses) other cells.

NEPHRITIS: Inflammation of the kidney.

NEUROSIS: A disorder of the mental constitution.

NEUTROPHIL: Granulated white blood cell.

NICONACID: Swiss-French trademark for a preparation of nicotinic acid.

NICOTINAMIDE (NIACINAMIDE): amide of 3-pyridinecarboxylic acid (niacin); its chemical formula is $C_6H_6N_2O$. A form of niacin.

NOXIOUS STIMULUS: Unpleasant or damaging substance or influence.

NUCLEOSIDE: One of four types of building blocks of DNA.

NUCLEUS: That part of a cell containing DNA.

PANTOTHENIC ACID: Constituent of the vitamin B complex.

PATHOGENIC: Producing disease or undesirable symptoms.

PATHOLOGIST: Expert in pathology.

PATHOLOGY: Branch of medicine that deals with changes in tissues or organs of the body caused by or causing disease.

PELLAGRA: Deficiency of niacin (one of the B vitamins) that causes diarrhea, dermatitis, and demential (loss of intellectual function).

PENICILLIN: Any of a large group of antibiotics.

PERIARTERITIS NODOSA: Form of vasculitis (inflammation of blood vessels) affecting small and medium-sized blood vessels; may be caused by hepatitis.

PERIPHERAL NEUROPATHY: Malfunction of nerves of the arms or legs.

PERNICIOUS ANEMIA: Condition caused by vitamin B12 deficiency and characterized by a reduction in red blood cells and spinal cord abnormalities.

PHAGOCYTE: Cell (macrophage, monocyte) that ingests other cells or debris.

PHAGOCYTOZED NUCLEAR MATERIAL: White cells that have ingested nuclei from other cells.

PHAGOCYTOSIS: Ingestion by phagocytes of foreign or other particles, or cells harmful to the body.

PHELBITIS: Inflammation of a vein.

PHOTOSENSITIVITY: Sensitivity to light energy.

PLACEBO: Inactive substance given to a patient either for its pleasing effect or as a control in experiments with an active drug.

PLASMA: Fluid portion of the blood in which the blood cells float.

PLASMA CELL: Tissue cell that makes antibodies.

PLEURISY (PLEURITIS): Inflammation of the membrane between the chest wall and the lung.

POLYARTERITIS: Same as periarteritis nodosa.

POLYARTHRITIS: Inflammation of several joints at the same time.

POLYMORPHONUCLEAR LEUKOCYTE: Same as neutrophil.

PREDNISONE: Chemical name for a synthetic steroid hormone.

PROGESTERONE: Female hormone produced during pregnancy that is primarily responsible for maintaining pregnancy and developing the mammary glands.

PROPERDIN: One of the complement proteins.

PROSTAGLANDIN: The prostaglandins are a large family of pharmacologically active lipids (fats) widely distributed in mammalian tissue.

PROTEINS: Building blocks of the body; regulators of cell function.

PROTEINURIA: Protein in the urine.

PSYCHOSOMATIC: Relationship of the body to the mind; having bodily symptoms from mental rather than physical disorder.

PTOSIS: Drooping of an eyelid.

PULMONARY: Pertaining to the lungs.

PUPILLARY REACTION: Constriction or dilation of the pupil of the eye in response to light.

PURPURA: Rupture of blood vessels with leakage of blood into the tissues.

RENAL: Pertaining to the kidneys.

RHEUMATOID ARTHRITIS: Chronic inflammatory disease of the joints.

SCLERODERMA: "Hard skin," a chronic connective tissue disease characterized by leathery thickening of the skin; the internal organs may also be involved.

SEDIMENTATION: Settling of red blood cells to the lower portion of a volume of blood that has been treated to prevent clotting.

SERUM: Blood from which cells and fibrin have been removed.

SERUM CREATININE LEVELS: Creatinine is a substance normally found in blood in low concentration, since it is eliminated from the serum by the kidneys; high serum creatinine levels indicate malfunction of the kidneys.

SERUM PROTEIN: Any protein in the serum.

SJÖGREN'S SYNDROME: Autoimmune disease characterized by dryness of the mouth and eyes.

SPONTANEOUS REMISSION: Marked improvement in a disease that occurs without medical intervention.

STREPTOCOCCUS: Bacterium that may cause sore throats (strep throat) and skin infections (erysipelas, scarlet fever) that may result in nephritis, inflammation of the kidneys, or rheumatic fever (inflammation of the heart and joints).

SUBACUTE CUTANEOUS LUPUS ERTHEMATOSUS: Lupus with characteristic skin lesions.

SULFADIAZINE: Antiinfective drug; one of the sulfonamides.

TESTIS: Synonym for testicle, the male reproductive organ responsible for production of sperm cells.

TETRACYCLINE: An antibiotic.

THERAPEUTICS: Study of the action of drugs and their application to the treatment of disease.

THERMAL BURNS: Injury to tissue caused by heat.

THROMBOCYTOPENIA: Reduction of circulating platelets.

THYROID GLAND: Gland located in the neck that produces thyroxine.

THYROIDITIS: Inflammation of the thyroid gland.

THYROXINE: Substance that affects the body's metabolic rate.

TITER: Highest dilution of a serum that gives a reaction with a substance.

T LYMPHOCYTE (T CELL): Lymphocyte involved in cellular immunity.

TOLERANCE TO NUCLEIC ACID ANTIGENS: Unresponsiveness to nucleic acids.

ULTRAVIOLET: Portion of the spectrum of sunlight that tans the skin.

UV-ALTERED DNA: DNA molecules disrupted by UV energy entering the cell, causing them to become antigen.

UV RADIATION: Radiation of energy of wavelengths 200 to 290 nm (UVC); 290 to 320 nm (UBV); 320 to 400 nm (UVA).

UREMIA: Marked kidney insufficiency characterized by nausea, vomiting, and even coma or convulsions, and a urine odor to the breath.

VASCULITIS: Inflammation of the blood vessels.

VASOMOTOR: Pertaining to control of the tone of the blood vessels; contraction of blood vessels causes blanching, whereas relaxation causes blushing.

VIRAL ETIOLOGY: Caused by a virus.

VIRAL PROTEIN: One of several constituents that make up a virus particle.

*Credit: Reprinted with permission of Charles Scribner's Sons, an imprint of Macmillan Publishing Company from IN SEARCH OF THE SUN by Henrietta Aladjem & Peter H. Schur, M.D. Copyright © 1972, 1988, Henrietta Aladjem and Peter H. Schur, M.D.

FOUNDATIONS

ALABAMA

LFA, Birmingham Chapter, Four Office Park Circle Ste. 302, Birmingham, AL 35223

LFA, Montgomery Chapter, P.O. Box 11507, Montgomery, AL 36111

ALASKA

LFA, Alaska Chapter, P.O. Box 211336, Anchorage, AK 99521-1336

ARIZONA

LFA, Greater Arizona Chapter, 2149 W. Indian School Road, Phoenix, AZ 85015

LFA, Southern Arizona Chapter, 3113 E. First St. Suite C, Tuscon, AZ 85716

ARKANSAS

LFA, Fort Smith Chapter, P.O. Box 10092, Fort Smith, AR 72917-0092

CALIFORNIA

LFA, Bay Area L.E. Foundation, 2635 No. First Street, Suite 206, San Jose, CA 95134

LFA, Southern California Chapter, 1101 South Robertson Blvd. Suite 208, Los Angeles, CA 90035

COLORADO

Lupus Foundation of Colorado, Villa Italia Offices, 7200 West Alameda, Lakewood, CO 80226

CONNECTICUT

LFA, Connecticut Chapter, 45 South Main Street, West Hartford, CT 06107-2402

DISTRICT OF COLUMBIA

Lupus Foundation of Greater Washington, 6210 No. Kings Hwy, Alexandria, VA 22303

FLORIDA

Dade/Broward Lupus Foundation, 2845 Aventura Blvd., No. Miami Beach, FL 33180

LFA, Brevard County Chapter, P.O. Box 372909, Satellite Beach, FL 32937

LFA, Florida Big Bend Chapter, 2108 Lytham Lane, Tallahassee, FL 32308

LFA, Palm Beach County Chapter, P.O. Box 18645, West Palm Beach, FL 33416

LFA, Pensacola Chapter, P.O. Box 17841, Pensacola, FL 32522-7841

LFA, Tampa Area Chapter, Village Center, 13232 North Dale Mabry Hwy, Tampa, FL 33618

LFA, Volusia Chapter, P.O. Box 1858, Daytona Beach, FL 32115

Lupus Foundation of Florida, 4706 Carmel Street, Orlando, FL 32808

LFA, North Florida Chapter, P.O. Box 10486, Jacksonville, FL 32247-0486

LFA, Suncoast Chapter, P.O. Box 23244, St. Petersburg, FL 33742

GEORGIA

LFA, Augusta Chapter, 4383 Ridge Point Dr., Augusta, GA 30909

LFA, Columbus Chapter, 233 12th Street, Suite 819, Columbus, GA 31901

LFA, Greater Atlanta Chapter, 2814 New Spring Road, Suite 102, Atlanta, GA 30339

LFA, Savannah Chapter, P.O. Box 2532, Savannah, GA 31402

HAWAII

Hawaii Lupus Foundation, 1200 College Walk Street Suite 114, Honolulu, HI 96817

ILLINOIS

LFA, Illinois Chapter, P.O. Box 42812-0812, Chicago, IL 60642

LFA, Danville Chapter, 322 East 13th Street, Danville, IL 61832

INDIANA

Indiana Lupus Foundation, 2701 East Southport Road, Indianapolis, IN 46227

LFA, Northeast Indiana Chapter, 5401 Keystone Drive Suite 202, Fort Wayne, IN 46825

LFA, Northwest Indiana Lupus Chapter, 3819 West 40th Avenue, Gary, IN 46408
IOWA
LFA, Iowa Chapter, P.O. Box 1723, Ames, IA 50010
KANSAS
LFA, Wichita Chapter, P.O. Box 16094, Wichita, KS 67216
KENTUCKY
Lupus Foundation of Kentuckiana, 2210 Goldsmith Lane #209, Louisville, KY 40218
LOUISIANA
Louisiana Lupus Foundation, 7732 Goodwood Blvd. #B, Baton Rouge, LA 70806
LFA, Cenla Chapter, P.O. Box 12565, Alexandria, LA 71315-2565
LFA, Northeast Louisiana Chapter, 102 Susan Drive, West Monroe, LA 71291
LFA, Shreveport Chapter, 1961 Bayou Drive, Shreveport, LA 71105
MAINE
Lupus Group of Maine, P.O. Box 8168, Portland, ME 04104
MARYLAND
Maryland Lupus Foundation, 12 W. 25th Street, Baltimore, MD 21218
MASSACHUSETTS
LFA, Massachusetts Chapter, 215 California Street, Newton, MA 02158
MICHIGAN
LFA, Michigan Lupus Foundation, 26202 Harper Ave., St. Clair Shores, MI 48081
MINNESOTA
LFA, Minnesota Chapter, 640 11th Avenue South, Hopkins, MN 55343
MISSISSIPPI
LFA, Mississippi Chapter, P.O. Box 24292, Jackson, MS 39225
MISSOURI
LFA, Kansas City Chapter, 10804 Fremont, Kansas City, MO 65807
LFA, Ozarks Chapter, 1814 West Katella, Springfield, MO 65807
LFA, Missouri Chapter, 8420 Delmar Blvd. #LL1, St. Louis, MO 63124
MONTANA
LFA, Montana Chapter, 3308 Lower River Road #40, Great Falls, MT 59405
NEBRASKA
LFA, Omaha Chapter, P.O. Box 14036, Omaha, NE 68124
LFA, Western Nebraska Chapter, P.O. Box 7, Gothenburg, NE 69138
NEVADA
LFA, Nevada Chapter, 1555 E. Flamingo Suite 439, Las Vegas, NV 89119
LFA, Northern Nevada Chapter, 480 Galletti Way #14, Sparks, NV 89431
NEW HAMPSHIRE
New Hampshire Lupus Foundation, c/o Ronald L. Calabraro, 14 Waterview Drive, Amherst, NH 03031
NEW JERSEY
LFA, South Jersey Chapter, P.O. Box 658, Cherry Hill, NJ 08034
Lupus Foundation of New Jersey, 287 Market Street, P.O. Box 320, Elmwood Park, NJ 07407
NEW MEXICO
LFA, Mexico Chapter, P.O. Box 35891, Albuquerque, NM 87176-5891
NEW YORK
LFA, Bronx Chapter, 1410 East Avenue 1F, Bronx, NY 10462
LFA, Central New York Chapter, Maria Regina Center Bldg. B, 1118 Court Street, Syracuse, NY 13208
LFA, Genessee Valley Chapter, P.O. Box 14614, Rochester, NY 14614
LFA, Long Island/Queens Chapter, 1602 Bellmore Ave., No. Bellmore, NY 11710
LFA, Marguerite Curri Chapter, P.O. Box 853, Utica, NY 13503
LFA, Northeastern NY Chapter, 126 State Street, Albany, NY 12207
LFA, Rockland/Orange County Chapter, 14 Kingston Drive, Spring Valley, NY 10977
LFA, Westchester Chapter, P.O. Box 133, Valhalla, NY 10595
LFA, Western New York Chapter, 205 Yorkshire Road, Tonawanda, NY 14150
New York Southern Tier Chapter, 19 Chenango Street, 410 Press Building,

Binghamton, NY 13901
LFA, SLE Foundation, 149 Madison Ave., New York, NY 10016
NORTH CAROLINA
LFA, Charlotte Chapter, 101 Colville Road, Charlotte, NC 28207
LFA, Raleigh Chapter, P.O. Box 10171, Raleigh, NC 27605
LFA, Western North Carolina Chapter, 339 Corbin Road, Franklin, NC 28734
LFA, Winston-Triad Lupus Chapter NCLF, 2841 Foxwood Lane, Winston Salem, NC 27103
OHIO
LFA, Akron Area Chapter, 942 N. main Street #23, Akron, OH 44310
LFA, Columbus Marcy Zitron Chapter, 5180 E. Main Street, Columbus, OH 43213
LFA, Greater Cleveland Chapter, P.O. Box 6506, Cleveland, OH 44101-1506
LFA, Northwest Ohio Lupus Chapter, 1615 Washington Ave., Findlay, OH 45840
LFA, Stark County Lupus Association, P.O. Box 1038, Massillon, OH 44648
OKLAHOMA
Oklahoma Lupus Association, 3131 N. MacArthur Suite 140D, Oklahoma City, OK 73122
PENNSYLVANIA
LFA, Lupus Alert, P.O. Box 8, Folsom, PA 19033
LFA, Delaware Valley Chapter, 44 W. Lancaster Ave., Ardmore, PA 19003
LFA, Northeast Pennsylvania Chapter, 417 Griffin Pond Road, Clarks Summit, PA 18411
LFA, Northwest Pennsylvania Chapter, P.O. Box 885, Erie, PA 16512-0885
LFA, Western Pennsylvania Chapter, 1323 Forbes Ave., Suite 200, Pittsburgh, PA 15219
Lupus Foundation of Philadelphia, 5415 Claridge Street, Philadelphia, PA 19124
Pennsylvania Lupus Foundation, P.O. box 264, Wayne, PA 19087-0264
RHODE ISLAND
LFA, Rhode Island Chapter, #8 Fallon Ave., Providence, RI 02908
SOUTH CAROLINA
LFA, South Carolina Chapter, P.O. Box 7511, Columbia, SC 29202
TENNESSEE
LFA, East Tennessee Chapter, 5612 Kingston Pike #5, Knoxville, TN 37919
LFA, Memphis Area Chapter, 3181 Poplar Ave. Suite 100, Memphis, TN 38111
LFA, Nashville Area Chapter, P.O. Box 481, Madison, TN 37116-0481
TEXAS
El Paso Lupus Association, 6145 Quail #504, El Paso, TX 79924
LFA, Dallas Chapter, Professional Plaza I Suite 211, One Medical Parkway, Dallas, TX 75234
LFA, Houston Chapter, 3100 Timmons Lane #410, Houston, TX 77027
San Antonio Lupus Foundation, McCullough Medical Center, 4118 McCullough Ave. #19, San Antonio, TX 78212-1968
UTAH
LFA, Utah Chapter, Inc., 385 24th Street #827, Ogden, UT 84401
VERMONT
LFA, Vermont Chapter, P.O. Box 209, South Barre, VT 05670
VIRGINIA
LFA, Central Virginia Chapter, P.O. Box 25418, Richmond, VA 23260-5418
LFA, Eastern Virginia Chapter, 735 Graydon Avenue, Norfolk, VA 23507
WEST VIRGINIA
LFA, Kanawha Valley Chapter, P.O. Box 8274, South Charleston, WV 25303
WISCONSIN
The Lupus Society of Wisconsin, 1568 So. 24th Street, Milwaukee, WI 53204
CFC OFFICE
Lupus Foundation of America, Federated Programs Office, 2510 Brentwood Blvd. Suite 304, St. Louis, MO 63144

AUSTRALIA
Arthritis Foundation of Queensland, P.O. Box 901, Toowong, Queensland 4066, Australia
Lupus Association of Tasmania, Inc., P.O. Box 404, Rosny Park, Tasmania, Australia 7018
Lupus/Scleroderma Group, Arthritis Foundation of Australia – SA, 99 Anzac Highway, Ashford, South Australia 5035
Victorian Lupus Association, Att: Enid Elton, Liaison, Box 811 F, G.P.O., Melbourne, Victoria, Australia 3001
The Lupus Assoc. of N.S.W., P.O. Box 271, Cammeray, New South Wales 2062, Australia
Riverina Lupus Support Group, 5 Pearson Street, Uranquinty, N.S.W. 2652, Australia

BELGIUM
Liga Voor Chronische Inflammatoire, Bindweefselziekten, Uitbreidingstraat 506, B - 2600 Berchem, Belgium

BERMUDA
The Lupus Association of Bermuda, P.O. Box DV 238, Devonshire, DV BX, Bermuda, Att: Debi Boorman

BRAZIL
Cristiano A. Zerbini, MD., 20 Chapel Street, Brookline, MA 02146

BULGARIA
LFA Chapter "Phillipopolis", Att: Dr. Emilie Spassova, 2 Yosif Shniter Street, 4000 Plovdiv, Bulgaria

CANADIAN PROVINCES — LUPUS FOUNDATION OF CANADA

CHINA
Zhang Xin, Chief – Dept. of Rheumatology, Xian Fifth Hospital, Xian City, Rhaanxi Province 710082, Peoples Republic, China

ENGLAND
"Rookery Nook", 17 Monkhams Drive, Woodford Green, Essex IG8 0LG
LUPUS U.K., Queens Court, 9 - 17 Eastern Road, ROMFORD, Essex. RM1 3NG
Luton & District Lupus Group, 19 High Mead, Luton, Beds., England LU3 1RY
Liverpool Lupus Group, 53 Westbourne Avenue, Thornton, Liverpool L2310P England

FRANCE
Association Francaise des Lupiques, 25 rue des Charmettes, 69100 Villeurbanne, France

GERMANY
Karin Hilmer, Lupus Erythematodes, Selbsthilfegemeinschaft e.v., Gollemkamp 3, 4600 Dortmund 15 Germany
Rheuma _ Ambulanz, Medizinische Universitats-Poliklinik, Wilhelmstr, 35-37, 5300 Bonn 1, Germany

HOLLAND
Nationale Vereniging, L.E. Patienten, Postbus 40, 1180 AA Amstelveen Holland

IRELAND
Lupus Support Group Ltd., 49 Killester Park, Dublin 5, Ireland
Hon. Sec. Cork Branch, 3 Ard na Greine, Evergreen Road, Cork 4 Ireland

ISRAEL
Israel Lupus Association, Harav Nissim 10, Raanana, Israel

ITALY
E di Immunologica Clinica, Ospedale S. Martino – XIII U.S.L., Viale Benedetto XV, 10, 16132 Genova, Italy
Clinica Dermatologica Universita, Policlinico-P., za Giulio Cesare, 70100 Bari, Italy

JAPAN
Kanazawa Medical University, Uchinada - Machi, Kahokugun, Ishikawa - Ken 920-02, Japan

MALAYSIA
Malaysian Society of Rheumatology, 26 Persiaran Jelutong, Damansara Heights, 50490 Kuala Lumpur, Malaysia, Att: Dr. Gek Liew Chin
MEXICO
Dr. J. Humberto Orozco-Medina, Coordinator "Club de Lupus Centro Medico de Occidente", Pedro Buzeta 870-B, 44660 Guadalajara, Jal., Mexico
NEW ZEALAND
Lupus Association of New Zealand, c/o Arthritis & Rheumatism Foundation of New Zealand, Inc., P.O. Box 10-020, Wellington, New Zealand
PHILIPPINES
Arthritis Foundation of the Philippines, Inc., Santo Tomas University Hospital, Espana Street, Manila, Philippines
POLAND
Instytut Reumatologiczny, Att: Dr. Henryka Maldykowa, ul. Spartanska 1, 02-637 Warszawa, Poland
PORTUGAL
Prof. Viana de Queiroz, Universidade de Lisboa, Hospital Universitario de Santa Maria, Av. Prof. Egas Moniz, 1699 Lisboa, Portugal
ROMANIA
CLINICA DERMATOLOGICA CLUJ-NAPOCA, str. Clinicilor nr. 3, 3400 Cluj-Napoca, Romania, Prof. Dr. Nicolae Maier, Chief of the Clinic
SCOTLAND
Strathclyde Lupus Group, Att: Mrs. Jane Elliott, 6 Hawkhead Road, Paisley, Scotland PA1 3NA
Fife, Lothian & Borders Lupus Group, c/o Mrs. Sue Pollock, 65 St. John's Drive, Dumferline, Fife, KY12 7TB, Scotland
SINGAPORE
Dr. Feng Pao Hsii, Vice Chairman, National Arthritis Foundation of Singapore, 336 Smith Street #06-302, New Bridge Centre, Singapore 0105
SPAIN
Spanish SLE Aid Group, Dept. of Internal Medicine - Unit 1, Hospital Clinic, Villarroel, 170, 08036 Barcelona, Spain, Dr. Joseph Font
SWEDEN
SLE-GRUPPEN 1 RMR, Solveig Karlsson, Bodavaegen 3, S-199 92 Enkoeping, Sweden
SWITZERLAND
Swiss Lupus Group, Gabriela Guenson, Beerenbachweg, 8555 Muellheim, Switzerland
WEST INDIES
Lupus Society of Trinidad & Tobago, c/o Skin Clinic, General Hospital, Charlotte Street, Port of Spain, Trinidad, West Indies